CUT THE CRAP

R *efined*

A *ddictive*

P *rocessed*

DEBORAH MORGAN
CUT THE CRAP!
& FIND YOUR PERFECT WEIGHT

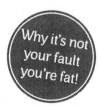
Why it's not your fault you're fat!

bookshaker

First Published In Great Britain 2011

by www.BookShaker.com

© Copyright Deborah Morgan

■ PRAISE FOR CUT THE CRAP

"I have lost over two and a half stone with this no nonsense weight loss plan and honestly, it was so easy. I had been struggling trying to lose the weight on my own for some time and getting nowhere, feeling quite despondent and frustrated. Deborah's programme has been so enjoyable. Almost instantly the weight started to fall off me and I felt so energised! I've had no cravings whatsoever. I have continued to socialise and even lost weight whilst on holiday, which was a first. I now feel amazing and have maintained my goal weight with no problem at all. The best thing of all is all the compliments I receive, I feel fantastic!"

ANNE WATSON

"For me, this programme has been nothing less than a miracle. When I eventually plucked up the courage to make the change, my health was of great concern. I suffered from diabetes type two, high cholesterol and my blood pressure was dangerously high. I was a walking time bomb. I have now lost over four stone and feel like a new person; I am enjoying a new lease of life. Within just a few weeks my blood sugars were normal and my blood pressure was lower than I can ever remember, Deborah's advice has literally saved my life! Thank you."

STUART HENDERSON

"Losing over two stone has been fantastic. My self esteem and confidence have increased, I wake up every day feeling light and energised! Once I learnt how the diet foods and constant dieting were making me fatter, I took Deborah's advice and embraced this natural alternative. The thing that has surprised me the most is how easy it's been. I never thought I could love fresh foods so much; my taste buds have totally changed and I know for certain I will never go back to my old ways. Why would I? I just love being slim! I feel so very proud of myself because I have maintained my weight now for over eight years... easy peezy."

KAREN NESFIELD

■ ACKNOWLEDGEMENTS

FIRSTLY, A HEARTFELT THANKS TO MY BEST FRIEND AND spiritual sister, Michele, who has been my health and spiritual mentor for the past 10 years. For introducing me to meditation, manuka honey and soya milk. For having faith in me and encouraging me all the way.

Thanks to my wonderful husband and life partner, Paul, who has also given me the support, encouragement and time out to write this book. For holding the fort whilst I was away and editing the reams of messy text I presented on my return.

Thank you to the Optimum Health institution in San Diego; it was a truly inspirational journey. For the hospitality and luxury of the Grand Hotel in Del Mar in San Diego, where I found a tranquil location to write. Thanks for the endless cups of peppermint tea and all the smiling faces.

Thank you to all the wonderful people and clients who have entrusted me with their goals and inspirations; they have been my greatest teachers.

And last but not least, a big thank you to all you wonderful friends who have eagerly awaited this book, with your encouragement, enthusiasm and love. It's finally here!

CONTENTS

Introduction 1

The most important thing you
will ever need to know 7

Pleasure not pain 23

Lies, lies and damned lies 35

Acid: the burning issue 47

Want to know the real reason you're fat? 61

Ditch the double act 69

Stress makes you fat too 75

Crap to cut 83

These are a few of my favourite things 127

You are what you drink 137

The power of exercise 141

Your personal transformation 151

Appendices 156

About the author 158

INTRODUCTION

"The poorest man would not part with health for money, but the richest would gladly part with all his money for health."
COLTON

Your path to freedom

CONGRATULATIONS! YOU'VE ALREADY TAKEN YOUR first big decision, not only to lose that unwanted weight, but also to improve your health and the quality of your life forever. Now, I'm sure this is not the first attempt you have made to win the "battle of the bulge". Like many people, including myself, you've probably spent what seems like most of your adult life searching for something that actually works for you. However, I am delighted to tell you that you have now finally found it. Follow my guidelines and this will be the final attempt you ever make to achieve the body you deserve and transform your life with new levels of energy and vitality.

Being a spiritual person, I believe there are no accidents in this universe. Everything happens for a reason. The very fact that you are reading this book is no accident. You were meant to. It's part of your destiny, and the timing is perfect. There's a saying, "When the student is ready, the teacher appears". Well, I am your teacher and you are my student. It's my privilege to be your guide and lead you down a path of discovery to your true, thinner, healthier and happier self.

Although I don't know you personally, I do care about you deeply. Helping other human beings transform their lives is my mission. Ever since my youth, I have been drawn to helping others. Indeed, every job I've had has been in the caring profession. Helping others nurtures my soul, and nothing makes me happier. In my personal life, my greatest friends and loved ones are people who were initially brought to me in a time of need. I seem to attract such people wherever I go.

I now know that you can't give to another without giving to yourself, so in a sense the pleasure is all mine anyway. For many years, I referred to myself as a "Transformational Therapist". Nowadays, I like to think of myself as a teacher. Some people refer to me as their life coach, others their therapist. Whatever the label, I help people change their lives, create outstanding health, prevent disease and generally live the life they deserve. I believe this is my gift, and my main purpose for being here on earth.

However this book made its way to you, whether it caught your eye at a bookstore or you heard about it from a friend, I just know you and I were meant to connect today. And I am so excited to reveal this permanent solution to your weight loss problems. In fact, I am bursting at the seams.

I have tried to keep the language as simple as possible, as I'm not in the business of baffling people with complicated words or boring scientific theories. Nice and easy, that's my philosophy. Everything in nature is simple and easy, and most of my teaching is based on Mother Nature's rules for life. These rely upon plain common sense and intuition, something we seemed to have become detached from. I would also like you to imagine that we're engaged in a conversation with each other. This way, you will absorb everything much more easily.

My programme has been born out of my own personal struggle with low self-esteem, weight issues and trying to find acceptance in society – all of which I have successfully conquered. It's not just about weight loss. It's also about something much more valuable: freedom. Once you have achieved your ideal weight, lost the surplus fat and are experiencing outstanding health, vitality and confidence every day, you are free to create the most compelling future. I call this my freedom programme; the term "weight loss plan" just doesn't do it justice.

In fact, many of the so called weight loss gurus and authors around today have never had a weight problem themselves. In my opinion, this means they're not equipped to write diet books and give advice. Many of the diets and diet aids you see endorsed by celebrities are done so because of a huge incentive called a cheque. This book has been titled *Cut The Crap* because that's exactly what you need to do if you want to normalise your body weight. The food conglomerates need to Cut The Crap, too. Which means they need to stop the lies and reveal the truth about what they're really putting in our foods, and why they are deliberately making us sick and fat.

Of course, in reality, the chances of them doing this are about as likely as me hang gliding to the moon. It would be like admitting manslaughter, so let's not bother going there. It took 50 years for the tobacco industry to be exposed, and it may take another 50 for the food and drug industry. You, however, can trust all the information I'm about to share with you. It's the truth, and if you open your mind and accept it, it will surely set you free. I wrote this book because I want to help as many people as possible free themselves from the shackles of dieting and the misery of being unhealthy and overweight.

In all honesty, I don't' believe anyone can enjoy life while they're feeling tired, fatigued, unhealthy and self-conscious every day of their lives. There is no such thing as being overweight and healthy, they are diametric opposites. When your body is healthy, it balances itself and weight loss is a natural occurrence. Excess weight is a symptom of poor health. And if you disagree, you are kidding and short changing yourself.

And why me?

You may be wondering what qualifies me to write about health and weight loss.

Good question. I have a wealth of experience in the health, wellness and fitness industry. Most important, I've also experienced the same low self-esteem, emptiness, frustrations, sadness, guilt, weakness and self-loathing as you, my friend. Yet not only have I turned my own life around, I've also helped thousands of others do the same.

I am not a doctor, nor a nutritionist. I am a person who is fascinated with the human body and passionate about nutrition and health. I am also someone who is increasingly angry and frustrated with the constant lies and brainwashing the food industry is delivering via the media. I also have two children, and am increasingly concerned about the welfare of theirs and future generations. If something doesn't change soon, I dread to imagine the consequences.

In addition, I have an overwhelming interest in spirituality, disease prevention and personal development. Growing up, I always wanted to be a doctor or a veterinary surgeon. One day my dreams were destroyed when an aunt took great delight in telling me "You need brains for that girl, you don't stand a chance!" Unfortunately, I believed her and my dreams were crushed in that very moment. I was 10 years old.

Still, as you can see, my fascination with the human body didn't stop there. My quest for knowledge has continued to this day. Anyone who knows me personally will tell you I am a "frustrated surgeon". I am a ferocious reader of medical research and psychology studies, plus anything about addictions, nutrition, spirituality and the anatomy of the human body. In my home, nutrition is the topic of conversation at almost every meal. We continually challenge one another with anatomy and nutrition quizzes! This is my way of teaching the kids and it works well. My home is crammed with the hundreds of books I've read over the past 16 years. My drawers are full of audio books, which I listen to at every opportunity.

With hindsight, I'm thankful I didn't take that formal medical training route and become a doctor. My knowledge has not come from dated textbooks, pharmaceutical companies or medical reps, but direct experience of people and life. I am able to think "outside the box" and bypass the brainwashing of conventional medicine. I have also watched and studied people for years, and witnessed the most transformational results when they change their diet and mindset.

By the way, the average GP has less than one day's training on nutrition, and very rarely updates it. Their job is to deal with illness, not to create health. And have you noticed how many GPs are overweight? Certainly not the right people to ask for advice on weight loss! In fact, I have had several GPs and surgeons as clients over recent years. They always confess to not knowing very much about nutrition, and compliment me on my wealth of knowledge. The majority of my clients are now referred by doctors, surgeons, dentists and other respected medical professionals, with the rest recommended by people who have successfully used my programme. I've always considered that if you want to be successful, study people who are already doing what you want to do. I am one of those people. I have successfully conquered my weight issue, and "walk the walk" every day of my life.

As I write this chapter, I'm sitting in the Canadian Rockies, overlooking the most spectacular, snow-covered mountains. The view is absolutely breathtaking and brings tears to my eyes. I am both excited and at peace. I feel close to my creator. It's at moments like this that my creativity comes alive. My stomach is fluttering and my heart pounding. I feel blessed to be given this opportunity to offer you the real solution to weight loss, health and vitality. In fact, I feel like I am the lucky one here! This programme is my gift to you, and I give it with love and blessings.

Energy is life's greatest gift. Without it, life has no meaning.

So that you can lose weight and, equally importantly, keep it off, I'm going to introduce you to a new approach that will literally change your life forever. You will learn how to enjoy your food and nourish your mind and body. You will discover how to eat without guilt. You'll find how to enjoy life and create outstanding health and energy, while at the same time losing weight easily.

In fact, the weight loss is actually going to be a positive side benefit of all the other wonderful changes you are about to experience. This unique approach will bring you the very best nutritional science available, which I have adapted over the past 10 years to create proven results. My research has taken me all over the world. I have studied the eating habits of different cultures, from the unhealthiest nations to the healthiest. I am a "people's person", so studying people is my ideal way of passing the day. Indeed, I have spoken to thousands of people on my journey, and put myself through all sorts of programmes. These have included fasting for five days, walking over hot coals, jumping off a telegraph pole and eating a raw and vegan diet for a month.

As well as studying what makes us fat, I have studied the eating and thinking habits of naturally slim people. I have combined these with what I believe is the most incredible health revelation available today – the "New Biology". The "Old Biology" was based on the findings of Louis Pasteur (1822-1895), who proved the germ theory of disease and invented pasteurisation. Yet we now know that germs do not create disease. Many people who have germs do not develop a disease. Rather, it is the condition of the host - your body - that determines whether or not a germ develops into a disease.

At one time, we all believed the world was flat, that patients with a fever should not be given water and that leeches cured illness. Now we know better because we have progressed and have new evidence and greater understanding. Through the use of high tech laboratories and microscopes, scientists today have been able to study the blood, giving us the information needed to substantiate the New Biology as scientific fact not hearsay.

Enjoy this philosophy, but, most of all, use it. In order to achieve the vibrancy you deserve, you must weave the information into the fabric of your life. Remember, physical health is the most important thing you can possess. Congratulations once again on having the courage to educate yourself and read this book. It's time now to get excited – and get cracking!

THE MOST IMPORTANT THING YOU WILL EVER NEED TO KNOW

"Insanity: doing the same thing over and over again and expecting different results."
ALBERT EINSTEIN

■ DIETS DON'T WORK. EVER!

Nobody ever said a truer word. We now have the biggest diet industry we've ever had, but just take a look at the figures below. How on earth could this happen if diets were any good?

Diets don't work and we all know it —at least, those of us who've been unfortunate enough to experience them. And that means an awful lot of people. Just ask yourself these questions – and be honest. I know it's hard, but acknowledging a problem is the first step to solving it.

> ➤ *How many diets have you been on?* The chances are it's a lot more than one. Which says it all, really.

> ➤ *Have you tried a variety of diets?* Which one was the most successful? And why did you do more than one diet anyway?

> ➤ *Did you reach your ideal weight?* If so, did you keep there for long? Or have you put all the weight back on again? In fact, are you heavier now than when you first tried to diet?

> ➤ *Have you actually enjoyed dieting?* Or does dieting just make you feel miserable and deprived?

By answering these questions honestly, the chances are you're starting to come to the conclusion that categorically diets don't work. If they did, you would only ever have to go on one. And you wouldn't be reading this book! Clearly, this is not the case.

■ A NATION OF PORKERS

➤ Around 44% of men and 33% of women in England are obese

➤ An additional 22% of men and 24% of women aged 16 or over in England were classified as obese (BMI 30kg/m2 or over)

➤ 38% of adults had a raised waist circumference in 2009 compared to 23% in 1993.

➤ Women were more likely than men (44% and 32% respectively) to have a raised waist circumference (over 88cm for women and over 102cm for men).

➤ In 2009, 16% of boys aged 2 -15 and 15% of girls were classed as obese, an increase from 11% and 12% respectively in 1995.

Taken from "Statistics on obesity, physical activity and diet: England 2011", a report by the NHS' Health and Social Care Information Centre, published February 2011.

There are over 25,000 diets currently on the market, with what seems like another fad diet appearing every month. The diet market is getting bigger along with our girths. In other words, there's more and more crap out there.

Yet even with more diets on the market, more diet foods, more information, more magazines, books and videos, as a nation we are still getting fatter. Surely, with all this information available we should have mastered the art of being eternally thin by now!

What amazes me is that man is the most intelligent species in the world and yet, along with our domesticated pets, we're the only ones who suffer obesity.

Astonishingly, almost every client I see tells me that they didn't have a weight issue until they started dieting. So could this mean that restricting your food intake and denying yourself your favorite foods switches on your 'fat making machine' and switches off your 'fat burning machine'?

Yes, yes, and **yes** again!

The truth is that dieting, eating man-made, chemical-laden diet foods and restricting your calorie intake messes up your metabolic rate. But don't panic. Providing you follow my advice, you can easily reset your metabolism and enjoy a healthy slim body while still eating the foods you love. I'm going to go into much greater detail on this later on. For now, though, just appreciate that no fad diet or diet aid is ever going to address the real cause of your weight problem.

Your weight is just a symptom, and simply treating the symptom is like pulling the weeds up in your garden and not expecting them to grow again. In other words, it's complete madness. To eradicate the symptom you need to find the cause and then the cause of the cause, the real root of the problem – more on this later.

Diets are designed to make you fat

As I've said, the diet industry is also getting bigger. It's now a booming, multi-billion pound industry that is cashing in on a growing epidemic. Yet is it doing anyone any good except the shareholders? Statistics now show that within a 12-month period, 95% of dieters put all the weight back on plus an extra two pounds.

So not only do diets not work, they also make you fatter. In fact, diet foods are designed to make you fatter. They are unsafe and cause all sorts of unpleasant side effects that we'll discuss later.

At some point on our journey through life, we've all succumbed to the lure of an advert that shows some miraculous, quick fix weight loss. Usually, it is a "before and after" photo that shows how some lucky person has transformed herself in the minimum time with minimum effort. What we don't see is the "after after" photos.

Quick fixes rarely work, not permanently anyway. There's a saying that what goes up must come down. Well, what goes up quickly must come down quickly too. And what comes off quickly must go back on quickly. The problem is, quick weight loss is mainly muscle and water loss, a little fat if you're lucky. The weight that goes back on is never muscle, just more fat, so fast results make you fatter and fatter.

If you are looking for a quick fix, then my programme is not for you. It's only for people who want long-lasting results. And I'd be interested to know why anyone would want anything temporary anyway. Would you like to be temporarily rich, or healthy for a month or so, or happy for a few weeks? Of course not. Yet diets and diet foods are temporary, so let's not go down that route. Let's go for gold and end the struggle once and for all.

Generally, people who eat diet foods were fat when they started and carry on getting fatter as they eat more and more: exactly what the diet industry wants. Some weren't even fat when they started, but just thought they were. Now after years of dieting, they have created a weight issue for themselves. That's unfortunate.

Am I convincing you about all this yet?

As you'll appreciate, when I use the word "diet'" I am not referring to a variety of foods that people are in the habit of consuming. Rather, it's used in the restrictive sense of "going on a diet", because this is what a diet is all about: restricting. It's about restricting your intake, removing your favorite food groups. This is why it makes you so miserable.

Almost all my clients view food as the enemy; they've got it so so wrong.

I believe that life is here to be enjoyed and that food is one of life's great pleasures. Unfortunately for most dieters, food becomes the enemy and the pleasure of eating is denied. And before we can go any further, you need to be totally convinced that **diets don't work**.

In order to make a permanent change, you need to **cut the crap** and break free from the habit of dieting for good. This is what actually causes the problem and gives you your weight issues. Once you break that habit you'll be able to reach your goal weight easily and effortlessly. And maintain it.

Diets simply create an unhealthy obsession with food — what we can't have we naturally want more of.

Denial always creates desire: deprive yourself of anything and eventually you will overeat or binge on it.

Where intention goes, energy flows

To lose weight permanently, you need to ditch the word "diet" from your everyday life. You need to stop thinking about it and talking about it. You have to stop searching for the next quick fix. Constantly being on a diet is making you focus on what you don't want to be: fat.

When you remove or restrict a food you enjoy, you feel you are genuinely making a sacrifice and so the food instantly becomes more precious. The more precious it becomes, the more deprived and miserable you feel — and the more you want it. This is what causes binge eating.

You must never remove foods you enjoy altogether. When you're overweight, you feel you've lost control of the foods you eat and the choices you make. When you "give in" to a food, overeat or binge, you are giving away your personal power. The result is a feeling of weakness and failure. And this goes for all addictions: smoking, alcohol, drugs, the lot.

To conquer your mental weakness, you need to reclaim your personal power and take back your self-control. Yet by focusing on dieting, you're constantly giving what you don't want more power. You need to move towards what you do want and give this your power instead.

There's a saying that runs, "Where intention goes, energy flows". This applies to everything in life. What we focus on becomes stronger and what we neglect becomes weaker. Not sure? Think about a time in your life when you have been driven and enthusiastic in order to achieve something, all you could think of was what you wanted. Did it come to fruition? Now think about something in your life you have neglected: maybe a relationship or an interest. Did this become weaker? Of course it did.

When couples fall in love, they often lose weight. When

brides prepare for their big day, they also often lose weight. When people start a new job or renovate a house, they often lose weight. And when people break up or go through a divorce they often lose weight. In fact, the weight seems to fall off without any conscious effort at all. Why is this? Is it the love, the divorce, the job that makes them lose weight? No, of course not. It's simply the fact that they become totally absorbed in something else and forget to focus on food, about what and when they eat. Food at this point in their life is not a consuming thought or habit, it's simply not a priority. In other words, they move their intention and focus away from it.

This is one of those universal laws that seem to work for anything, especially your weight issue. By constantly worrying, talking and thinking about your weight and weighing yourself daily, you're putting all your attention on the problem that you actually want to move away from. You're giving the fat the power to grow.

All this focusing on not having the "real version" simply makes you want and eat more food than ever. And, God knows, if anybody appreciates this it's me. I used to buy all those nonsense low fat, low sugar biscuits and stuff. They tasted like cardboard and were totally unsatisfying. In fact, they were total crap. Yet because I thought I was being "good", I used to eat the whole packet. No wonder I was fat.

Off their trolley

Next time you're in the supermarket, find a few overweight people. See what's in their shopping trolley. Chances are you'll find low fat, reduced fat, reduced sugar and diet foods. You'll also see stuff like highly fattening chocolates and cakes. Just who are they kidding?

Just knowing you're buying something that says "reduced" on the packet makes you feel fat and deprived. Yet again you're reminding yourself that you are not "allowed" the real thing. All this does is create desire and eventually you will overeat on all the fattening foods you've deprived yourself of – on top of all the substitute foods you've also bought.

···➤ *What we focus on becomes stronger.*
What we neglect becomes weaker.

Think like a man

From my work as a therapist, I've noticed this is more of a female thing. Men, thankfully, don't buy into the diet food hype in quite the same way. Someone once told me many years ago, "If you want to be slim, think like a man". Before a man sits down for his evening meal, he doesn't work out how many calories, points, sins or carbohydrates he's had that day. Nor does he analyse the calorie content of the meal he's about to eat. He just enjoys his food. He has what he fancies and what his body needs. There's something to be said for this way of thinking, and it's exactly how I want you to be too.

Men tend not to pick between meals, either. That's because they satisfy themselves at meal times. They eat what they want, not what someone else tells them they should have. Being on a diet feels like you are being told what to do, and no one likes that.

···➤ *Little pickers wear big knickers!*

Find your focus

Throughout this book, I'm going to ask you to turn your back and neglect what you don't want and nurture and nourish what you do want, both mentally and physically. Together, we're going to starve that extra weight of all your attention. We're going to nourish your physical body with delicious foods that create what you're really looking for – health, energy and a slender body.

I use this method all the time when looking for a parking space. Before I set off, I focus powerfully on a vacant space in front of the place I want to visit. It works for me practically every time. Great fun with the kids, too. Try it yourself

Sadly, the majority of people spend their lives running away from what they don't want and never move towards what they do want. They spend all their time complaining and being unhappy. They dwell constantly on their negative relationship with food. This is how dieting affects you in the long run. You spend your time looking for the latest quick fix, beating yourself up, counting the calories, talking about it, thinking about it constantly. That's why you get stuck. You give the very thing you want to move away from more power. That's why the problem just gets worse and worse.

Think of the weight you were when you first began to diet. Now think of how many diets you have tried, and how much thought and effort you have wasted only to end up heavier than you were when you started. Ask yourself, what else you would keep doing without getting results? What else would you keep doing that you knew was going to end up making the situation worse? (OK, you didn't know this before, but you do now.)

Think positively

To achieve long-lasting results, you need to know exactly where you are going and what you want. You need to be clear in your mind to reach your goal weight. If you constantly feel bad about your body, this is a powerful negative feeling; you'll never be able to change your body if you're always finding fault, all this will do is attract more weight.

Take a few minutes to think about all the things about yourself that are good, all the things that people like about you. As you think these positive thoughts and begin to feel good about yourself, you begin to prepare yourself for achieving your perfect weight..

You can't possibly begin to make changes for the better from a place of self-criticism - you need to come from a place of love. We are all like human transmission towers, transmitting frequencies with our thoughts. If you want to change anything in your life, you need to change the frequency by changing your thoughts.

It's a bit like tuning into a different radio station. Your thoughts shape and form your life. Every thought you have ever had has brought you to the point in your life you're at now. If you want to create a better life you need to start focusing on better thoughts. Thoughts are feelings and the quality of your life ultimately depends on how you feel about yourself.

In my practice, I am often saddened by the way clients describe themselves. They constantly say things like "I'm too fat", "I'm too thin, too ugly, too old, too stupid, too gross, too weak…" When I ask them who else shares the same opinion or has given them this label, they usually say, "No one, just me".

This perpetual negativity creates a lifetime of unhappiness. In almost every case these labels are nonsense. The first thing I ask my clients to do is to bin the self-criticism, the name-calling and the perpetual negative self-talk. Instead, I ask them to say something nice about themselves every time they go past a mirror. Although initially this may seem a bit weird, within a few short days their self-esteem is on the up and they are feeling much better. Nothing good ever came from negative self-talk, but great things always come from the positive stuff.

···➤ *Living in the past is like driving using the rear view mirror. You don't get very far.*

■ MIRROR, MIRROR ON THE WALL

Here's a wonderful exercise I still use myself from time to time. If you have any issues with negative self-talk and self-criticism, I strongly recommend you practise it daily. It may feel bizarre at first, but do it anyway.

- ➤ Stand in front of a mirror, look into your eyes and say "I love you, I love you, I really love you".
- ➤ Do it first thing in the morning, last thing at night and often during the day.
- ➤ If uncomfortable feelings come up, feel them and let them pass through, then repeat "I love you, I really love you".
- ➤ Forgive other people in the mirror too. Use it to talk to them. Tell them the things you're afraid to in person, like you want their love and approval.

···➤ *Forgiveness sets you free.*

You simply must try the mirror work. It's a very liberating experience. Forgiveness sets you free. It removes the burden of guilt and shame and has been one of the most powerful healing experiences of my life. And when you do it consistently, you can make great changes in less than a month.

If you are an emotional eater, there's a good chance you are hurting. It may not be on the surface, but somewhere deep inside. When we experience emotional pain on a deep level we often reach out for the comfort of food to escape. Yet diets will never address these issues. You need to go deeper and do some self-healing. Emotions are like messages, knocking on the door of your heart. Ignore them and they knock louder and louder until you eventually let them in. If you do have emotional issues, I would seriously suggest seeking professional help.

In truth, this is a subject very close to my heart. I go into more detail on my own issues later on, but for now I'll just say this: for 38 years I carried the burden of grief, guilt, shame and rejection. My parents died when I was young and I was never given the chance to go to their funeral, or even to grieve properly. The day my father died we had had a huge row. He had made me some freshly squeezed orange juice for breakfast and buttered the toast on the same cutting board as he had placed the orange pieces.

As a moody teenager I refused to eat the soggy toast and left for school. As I stood at the bus stop with my friends, my father ran behind me with a new piece of toast. Highly embarrassed, I shouted at him and threw the toast back. He suffered from angina and had a heart attack later on that same day whilst I was at school. He died alone, on a bus.

To this day I will never know what caused his heart attack and have lived with the anguish ever since.

I never got the chance to say goodbye or tell him how much I loved him. Having moody teenagers of my own who refuse to eat breakfast has helped me, but it still hurts deeply.

I buried my grief and guilt deep inside and my life was

very unhappy. I coped by overeating, abusing my body and self-criticising. Yet all the time I was sabotaging my own life unknowingly. It was only when I began to work on my inner child, to forgive myself and accept that I was not to blame, that I was able to release the negativity and experience the joy of life.

If you would like to know more about the ways you can heal from the inside, I recommend you read a wonderful book called *You Can Heal Your Life* by Louise L. Hay. It was a book that helped me heal and changed my life for the better.

Give yourself the power

People who get places in life do so because they know where they want to go to. It's all about clarity of purpose. Essentially, clarity is power. Once you're clear on what you want, you have the power to achieve anything you want in your life.

I don't mean just telling yourself, "I want to lose weight" or "I wish I wasn't so fat". That won't give you clarity or power. To create power you need to look at the things that motivate you to lose weight and the real reasons you want to be slim. This is your outcome.

It's the way you want to feel when you have lost all the weight. Realise that losing weight is only the process that gets you to your goal. It's a means to the end, not the end in itself. It's the end you need to focus on. This is what will give your life much greater meaning.

For some people, it's simply vanity: being able to wear more fashionable clothes; getting wolf-whistles walking down the high street; turning heads when you walk into a bar. All that sort of stuff, and why not?

For others, it's being around to watch their children and grandchildren grow up; or taking back their lost health and fitness. For me it was self-esteem and confidence – I needed more of it.

In truth, any reason is a great reason as long as it's yours. It's impossible to be motivated by someone else's goal. The motivation has to come from you.

Another key point to grasp is that to make changes it helps to be uncomfortable with where you are at right now. A comfortable place is often not the best place to make changes from.

What floats your boat?

We're all different. It's vital to find out what's driving you.

a) Your 'Away' motivators
➤ **List on a piece of paper, in order, the five most important reasons why you must lose weight. These are all the negative feelings you no longer want to feel.**

b) Your 'Towards' motivators
➤ **Now list the top five reasons why you want to be slim. These are the positive feelings you want to experience every day.**

Congratulations! You've just clarified the real reasons why you want to lose weight. You've also revealed the negative feelings you want to move away from. Most important, you've uncovered all the empowering feelings you are moving towards. These will trigger the changes you'll make for the rest of your life.

Weight loss will be one of the most positive experiences you'll have and it's vital to keep your goals in front of you at all times. See why to simply say "I want to lose weight" isn't enough now? Admit it. How many times have you said that to yourself! And where did it get you? Exactly!

You need to know and understand why you feel as you do. And the reasons must be personal to you if they are to be life-changing. This is how you achieve emotional leverage – "The Golden Key" to your freedom!

If you take my advice, you'll make a copy of this list and put it somewhere where you can read it every day. Remember, repetition is the mother of all skills. The more you reinforce yourself, the easier your journey to a slender body and better health.

We're not quite finished with that pen yet. Now close your

eyes and imagine yourself at your ideal weight. Then describe, in as much detail as you can, the difference it will make to your everyday life and the way you feel. Describe in detail how you look, imagine you are looking through the eyes of someone who loves you dearly. Imagine the words they would use to describe you and write them all down.

Feels good doesn't it? At this point, I suggest you buy a personal journal. It's ideal for setting goals, developing strategy, creating "leverage" and reviewing progress.

Get real

As we've seen, just focusing on the weight loss is no good because it's only the process; you need to concentrate on the outcome. You need to imagine how good you will feel and how much more enjoyable life will be when you're slim. These feelings of pleasure will empower you and strengthen your willpower and motivation.

So far, so good? Well, now I'm going to ask you to imagine what your life will be like if you don't lose the weight as well. It may seem like a bummer, but nobody ever solved a problem by not facing up to it. So just beat yourself up a little. It will be worth it, trust me. It will be the last time, I promise.

Over the past few years, you've been getting heavier and heavier, so it's very likely you'll get even fatter in future. Close your eyes and imagine yourself in five years time with another stone or two around you. Try asking yourself these questions:

> ➤ How will you be feeling, healthwise?
> ➤ What will it do to your self-esteem and confidence?
> ➤ How about your relationships – for example, will you enjoy intimacy? Do you enjoy intimacy now?
> ➤ What sort of clothes would you be wearing?
> ➤ Would you feel proud or ashamed of your body?

Take your time here, and let the answers come at their own pace. Allow your emotions to surface. Imagine the misery you would experience every day if you had not made the change.

Focusing on the pain will empower you as well. This process of visualisation is very effective.

You have a disease. You're fat!

You must realise that the excess weight you're carrying crept up on you slowly. That's why you got comfortable with it. Yet just try imagining that one morning you woke up, suddenly two stones heavier. Your joints are aching. You're tired and breathless. You feel bloated and cumbersome. How would you react? You'd probably panic and think you'd contracted a dreaded disease.

Well, in truth you have. It's called being fat!

It's the same disease that's been creeping up on you slowly all these years and you've just got used to it. With every half stone you've gained you've probably simply raised the bar and kidded yourself it's an acceptable weight.

At one time in your life, being just 7lbs overweight would have been unacceptable. But then you got used to that and thought nothing of it. Then you let another stone go on, and got used to that. Then two stone. See where we're going here?

Make no mistake. Being fat is not only unsightly. It's a threat to your health. It affects you both mentally and physically. It prevents you from enjoying life the way you deserve to.

You must now decide what weight gain is unacceptable, and what weight you want to be. Then make it happen. And don't be put off. Together, we'll make this weight loss journey easy and enjoyable. You do, however, have to decide what you want to lose. Do you want to lose 10lbs of muscle? 10lbs of water? Or 10lbs of fat?

When people tell me "I want to lose weight", I ask them what kind of weight? They usually have to think about it before they say, "Fat, of course". "Good" I say, "because it's the only type of weight you will lose using this programme". You need to be very clear in your mind that your sole aim is to burn fat and build muscle. There, now that's sorted out, let's move on swiftly.

More reasons why diets don't work

Diets usually result in short term loss and long term gain. Every diet leaves you heavier than the one before did – by 2lbs on average.

They screw up your hypothalamus, the gland that controls your metabolic rate and appetite.

They make you feel hungry and lethargic.

When the weight goes back on it's not as muscle but fat, which means you end up fatter than when you started. The lower your muscle mass, the lower your metabolic rate.

They slow down your metabolic rate by sending false alarm signals to the body to preserve energy rather than burn it.

They can slow down weight loss so much that you become "metabolically resistant". Your metabolic rate goes into hibernation, causing weight gain and lethargy.

They lead to malnutrition, creating weak immune, skeletal and nervous systems, together with weak eyes. Every overweight person suffers from malnutrition.

Lack of minerals causes the body to tap into its reserves, robbing calcium from the bones and magnesium for our muscles –the reason why middle-aged women become flabby and suffer from brittle bones.

Yo-yo dieting results in poor muscle tone.

Altogether, diets make you feel crap. So cut them out!

For even more reason, just look at the first three letters – "Die".

That says it all, really!

···➤ *The less you eat, the longer you live.*

PLEASURE
NOT PAIN

HAS WEIGHT LOSS BEEN A PARTICULARLY PAINFUL process for you in the past? Has it left you feeling deprived, uncomfortable, hungry or irritable? Then no wonder you failed; who in their right mind would put themselves through all this voluntarily?

And once you bowed to the inevitable, caved in and fell off the diet, no doubt you then felt like a failure. Over time, you started to associate losing weight with discomfort and all the other negatives. Repeating this process time and time again, as many dieters do, only perpetuates feelings of weakness and low self-esteem. These feelings become logged in your memory bank and the subconscious associates them with weight loss.

So now, every time you think about losing weight, your subconscious relates this to a negative feeling and does anything it can to prevent you even trying, never mind succeeding. Most people would recognise this as "lack of willpower" or the inability to get motivated. If the subconscious mind, the driving part of your mind, associates pain with change, it will do anything it can to avoid it and weight loss will be difficult, if not impossible. Remember, the number one priority of your subconscious is self-protection and it will act appropriately.

Now the good news! My approach does not rely on immense willpower or positive thinking. Rather, it's all about

> ➤ Linking pleasure to where you really want to be in life.
> ➤ Creating feelings of joy and happiness.
> ➤ Focusing on what your body needs.
> ➤ Reminding yourself of the way it feels to be slim and healthy, something many dieters have become totally removed from.

➤ Reconnecting with your mind and body, and becoming much more alert and aware.

➤ Tuning in to your natural instincts, desires and intuitions, and ignoring the external prompts and constant brainwashing the food industry bombards you with.

➤ Listening to Mother Nature.

➤ Applying common sense.

➤ Remembering you don't have to do this, you get to do it.

If you embrace this program it will be easy.

···➤ *You will never rise above the opinion you have of yourself.*

It's the journey, not the destination

More than anything else, to lose weight permanently you need to attach feelings of pleasure to the process. This is the "golden key" we call leverage. Weight loss can be a beautiful and liberating experience, provided you programme your mind for pleasure rather than pain.

In this programme there are no failures. Success is found in the journey itself, not the destination. Your aim is to feel good every day, to enjoy delicious foods, to have bundles of energy, increased confidence and self-esteem and, most importantly, outstanding health. I want you to squeeze the juice out of life and live for the moment.

Far too many people are simply waiting for the "magic moment" when they lose the weight, get the rise, meet their soul mate, retire or achieve something spectacular that will make them happy. Get it straight now: if you live this way, you will never experience happiness in this lifetime. If you live in the future, you miss the moment.

Happiness is our birthright and you can have it right now, if you choose to. There's a magic moment to have today if you want it. It's all about your mind-set. The Buddhists say that every morning you should imagine today is your last day on earth and decide how you would like to spend it. After all, whatever it is you want to do, why wait until your last day to do it? Do it today and experience the joy of life now. To repeat, success is the journey not the destination, and my aim is to help you to enjoy your journey by experiencing health, freedom and vitality every single day. Life certainly feels much better when you have the energy to enjoy it. What's more, laughter attracts joy, releases negativity and leads to miraculous cures.

····➤ *Live every day with an attitude of gratitude!*

No's are no-no's

With me there are no rules – rules are just there to be broken. There are no forbidden foods, no "good" or "bad" foods. Instead, there are simply recommendations about what to eat and what to avoid. You are an adult, you decide when and what you eat, simple as that.

There is no weighing or measuring, and no calorie counting. There are no "points", or "sins" to beat yourself up over. In fact, there's no berating or ridicule at all, just encouragement and love. Now you can resign from the self-beaters club.

Up until now, you've most probably been trying to act like a tall tree, with your roots firmly in the ground yet no room for movement. Instead, I want you to imagine yourself like the seaweed on the bottom of the ocean. I want you to "go with the flow" and take a relaxed approach to weight loss. Give yourself a well-earned break. Being strict with yourself is like being back at school.

If you start off with rules and rigidity, you're setting yourself up for failure before you even begin. No person on this earth can remain rigid for the rest of his or her life. How many times have you started a diet determined to succeed, only to knock it on the head in just a few days? In my own case, it would be just a few hours! When you lead a busy life and have to use willpower to look after the children, manage the house, go to work, visit the gym etc, no matter how determined you are, your willpower fades away over time. And that's exactly my point.

Using willpower alone just doesn't work. You use willpower in every other area of your life, and when it comes to yourself there's usually none left.

All I ask is for you to have an open mind, be kind to yourself, love your body and nourish it with positive thoughts and nutritious foods. Above all, drop the need to be a perfectionist. There's no such thing as perfection. If you aim for perfection you're just setting yourself up for failure. The very first time you "weaken", even a little, you will feel that you've failed and throw in the towel. After all, how many times have you done that already? It's why you are still here, trapped in a body that feels uncomfortable and unloved.

···➤ *Aim for progress, not perfection.*

Honesty is the only policy

I simply can't over emphasise it: settling for being overweight is settling for second best in life. If you settle for less than you know you can have, you are not being fair or honest with yourself. What's more, it can cause a lifetime of turmoil and unhappiness. If what you see in the mirror doesn't reflect your true soul then you owe it to yourself to raise your standards and create a healthy body you can feel proud of.

At the end of the day, it's how you feel about yourself that matters. You don't have to ask anyone else "Do I look fat in this?" or "Do I need to lose weight?" You know the answers already, don't you? In my experience, loved ones will never tell you they think you look fat. Really, how could they? They love you and know the truth would hurt you. In turn, this would only hurt them so they tell a white lie to make you feel better.

In truth, it's unfair to ask anyone else whether you need to lose weight. Who are you kidding, relying on other people's opinions anyway? If you were happy with yourself, you wouldn't have to ask the question in the first place. I am brutally honest with my clients and they usually end up in tears. The tears usually come from a realisation that they have been lying to themselves. If you want to know if you are fat and need to lose weight, just do the simple exercise described here. It takes courage but it really works so I urge you to do it.

Are you one of these people who avoid having photos taken? Being an ostrich will never solve your problem; avoidance is denial. It's time now to face the truth and deal with it. You have let your body get out of shape and now you're taking back control.

■ THE BARE TRUTH

> - Stand in front of a mirror totally naked.
> - Relax every muscle, and don't suck your stomach in!
> - Take a good long look at yourself from every angle.
> - Do you like what you see? Do you find yourself attractive and sexy?
> - Would you feel comfortable putting a bathing suit on and parading in front of your ten closest friends?
> - Would your partner/spouse still fancy you if you met each other today for the first time?

Many of my clients haven't looked at themselves in a full-length mirror for years. No wonder they've got fatter; denial is disastrous. To make changes, you need to accept where you are right now and stop kidding yourself. If you are comfortable with yourself, you will never change. You need to feel pain to create leverage.

There's a phrase that goes, "We even get comfortable in what we are uncomfortable with". It's very true. I remember when I first did the mirror exercise, I asked my ex-husband to take a photograph of me. He resisted at first because he knew the outcome would be painful for both of us. Eventually, after pleading with him, he reluctantly agreed. That evening I cried myself to sleep and I knew something had to change. I kept the photo, though, and still have it hidden away somewhere. It's a reminder of how I will never be again.

It may seem a tall order right now, but I know that if you implement the changes in this programme you will be able to achieve your goals easily and effortlessly. Just remember to take baby steps. Go slowly and reward yourself along the way.

Fast is slow and slow is fast

It may sound odd, but the slower you work through this programme, the faster you will get results. On the other hand, if you rush it, your weight loss will be slower. So be realistic when setting your target weight, as an unrealistic goal will always end up as failure. It's a good idea to choose a weight you have comfortably maintained for over six months in the past.

Your target weight is not dependent on the charts, on what your doctor tells you or even on your previous weight. When you can stand in front of the mirror butt naked and like what you see, you've reached your goal weight – simple as that.

Make sure you record your starting weight, and review it weekly. A "before" photo will help you. I recommend you weigh yourself once a week, preferably mid-week. Do it first thing in the morning, and butt naked. Monitoring your success is crucial and the rewards will make your journey a pleasure. You won't always lose weight, but the main thing is to make sure you don't gain any.

If you would like to see a picture of yourself at your ideal weight I offer a service called Body Imaging, which is available on my website. Many people tell me they can't imagine themselves at their target weight, but visualisation is important for goal setting and this service helps you. It's very easy: you email me a picture of you at your present weight and let me know your target weight and the areas of your body you are most concerned with. I need a few more details such as age, height etc., and then the magic happens. Within a few days you will receive an image of you at your ideal weight; you can see the difference before your very eyes! The picture is very empowering and motivating and will help you keep your goals in front of you at all times.

···➤ *The past is history, the future's a mystery and today is a gift. That's why it's called the present.*

The power of positive affirmations

An affirmation is simply a group of words or a saying that you repeat over and over again to enlist your subconscious mind in support of your goals. By saying these words repeatedly, you access the subconscious mind, penetrating it with new positive feelings and making the changes you want easier. You also attach real belief to the words, and visualise your end goal. This emotion makes words become very powerful. Mind and body become aligned with each other, motivating you to succeed. Successful people do this all the time, with or without knowing. They believe in themselves constantly and have an inner knowledge that they will succeed. They never focus on the failure they don't want, rather they have a burning desire within them that ultimately makes success inevitable.

The book Think and Grow Rich by Napoleon Hill has been a best seller since 1934 and is based on 20 years' research of the richest and most successful people in the world. The one thing Hill found all these people had in common was that they used both mental and verbal affirmations to secure their success. They never allowed doubt to hinder or block their progress. Instead, they fueled the burning desire within them with positive daily affirmations.

Sadly, when dealing with weight issues most of us do the opposite. We bombard ourselves with negative daily affirmations such as:

"I'll never be slim"
"Why am I so fat?"
"I always have to diet"
"I can't eat anything without putting on weight"
"I hate my body"
"I'll always be this way"
"I've been fat since I was a child"
"I have a slow metabolic rate"

Logically enough, this perpetual destructive self-talk is known as "negative affirmation". This can also penetrate the subconscious mind, which starts to work against you. You then get stuck, no matter how hard you try.

Whatever the diet, if your internal belief is focusing on what you don't want, then this is what the subconscious believes and keeps moving towards.

Although we consciously want so desperately to lose weight, many of us constantly brainwash the subconscious mind with negative thoughts. These merely confuse us and prevent our goals being a reality. To deal with this, I use a method called "Cancel Cancel". I learnt this many years ago and it's very powerful.

Here's how it works. Every time you hear yourself thinking a negative thought or saying a negative word, immediately say the word "Cancel". Most of the time, the thought pops up again, a bit like when you close your computer down: first you tell it to shut down, then a few seconds later another sign pops up and says "Are you sure?" Irritating, isn't it? Well, the brain works the same way, so you need to say "Cancel, cancel" and then change your thought to a more positive and empowering one right away.

In reality, this habit of negative self-talk is like going one step forward and two steps backwards. You get nowhere fast. To achieve success you need congruency of both your minds. In other words, the conscious and subconscious need to be in full agreement with each other. If in one breath you are saying, "I desperately want to lose weight" and in the next you come out with "I'll always be fat", you create incongruence and confusion in the mind. It is literally a battle of the minds, and as the subconscious is the strongest part of the mind, the thought that penetrates this area will always be the dominating factor.

Remember, "Clarity is power". Wanting to lose weight but not having the belief is like having a Ferrari on the drive without an engine. Again, you won't get very far. This explains why dieting alone doesn't work, and why people experience cravings, withdrawal, weakness and failure.

You probably know someone who eats like a horse, and they proudly declare "I can eat whatever I want and I'm always my perfect weight."". And so the genie of your subconscious says "Your wish is my command!" You probably also know someone who, conversely, says, "I can't eat anything without gaining weight". And so once again the genie grants their wish. Your subconscious is surprisingly good at doing what it's told.

Again, the solution is simple. Change the way you think and you change your metabolic rate. It's been proven time and time again. You can change your physiology just by changing your thoughts.

···➤ *Change the way you look at things and the things you look at change.*

What you think, you become

I know this to be true from firsthand experience. Indeed, I have personally walked over burning hot coals six times during the last nine years. Several of my friends and clients have literally followed in my footsteps. And these coals are burning – no, I mean really burning! Somewhere between 750 to 1,000 degrees centigrade; enough to burn off your bones, never mind your feet. Yet by conditioning our minds and changing the biochemistry of our bodies, we were able to walk across the coals without a single burn. Now, that is how powerful the human mind is!

This amazing feat was accomplished not by using any props or protective footwear, but simply by choosing thoughts that did not relate to heat, fire or burns. Several years ago, I took my wonderful friend Fiona along. She suffers from diabetes type one and has nerve damage to her feet. If she had burnt her feet the consequences would have been disastrous, yet she also did the walk burn-free. I took my husband, Paul, with me recently. He was a firefighter for 16 years and, as you can imagine, was extremely cautious and respectful of fire. When he did this, along with around 10,000 other apprehensive people, his life changed in that very moment. Now he knows he can accomplish anything he wants, providing he puts himself in a suitably positive powerful mindset.

In truth, it's not really about the walking over coals. They are just a metaphor for life and how you can access your personal power and alter your physiology simply by changing your thoughts.

Norman Vincent Peale said, "Change your thoughts and you change your life". The same applies to your body. You can achieve anything you want, as long as you believe it. You can slow down the ageing process, prevent illness and disease, speed up or slow down your metabolic rate and, of course, lose weight.

So the answer is, what you want, you must think. First, you need to decide exactly what it is you want, why you want it and what pleasure it will bring to your everyday life. Then you need to feed your subconscious mind with daily positive affirmations to create the motivation and inner belief to achieve your goals.

■ GET PERSONAL

To be effective, affirmations should always have the four Ps. In other words, they should be:

➤ **Positive**
➤ **Personal**
➤ **Powerful**
➤ **Present tense**

Here are some affirmations I love and use personally on a daily basis:

"Every day I get slimmer and slimmer"
"Every day I get healthier and healthier"
"Every day in every way I become more and more successful"
"I deserve the best and I accept the best now!"

With affirmations, some times of day are better than others. I've found that the best times are first thing in the morning, last thing at night, and when walking, exercising or driving. Indeed, I love shouting them out in my car and people just assume I'm singing!

In his book *The Master Key System*, Charles Haanel claims that there is an affirmation that incorporates every single thing that a human being can ever want. He also considers that affirmation will bring about harmonious conditions to all things, adding:

"The reason for this is because the affirmation is in strict accordance with the truth, and when the truth appears every form of error or discord must necessarily disappear."

If you like the sound of this, the affirmation is:

"I am whole, perfect, strong, powerful, loving, harmonious and happy"

Try it now and see how you feel when saying these supremely positive words. The key is to visualise your goal as you say the words out loud. If you can shout them out loud then so much the better. Whatever the volume, the key thing is to do it with gusto and belief. The more emotion and belief you attach, the more impact the words will have on your subconscious mind. Remember, when it comes to eating habits our subconscious mind is the big boss.

It's time now to get moving, so get excited and go for it! It's important, however, that you read each chapter of this book thoroughly and don't skip any.

I have taken great care in putting it together to bring you the maximum benefit of my experience, so bear with me. There is no fast track, and no short cuts. You need to understand it all to get the desired results. So, however long it takes for you to read this book - a week, two weeks or maybe a month – it's a small price to pay for something that is going to change the rest of your life.

LIES, LIES AND DAMNED LIES

OUR BODIES ARE REALLY JUST A SKELETON COVERED with yesterday's food.

It's true. Our bodies haven't changed much, if at all, for thousands of years. Yet the food we eat today is nothing like the stuff we were eating even just 40 years ago! This fact alone tells me something's going wrong. Big time.

We developed to eat a naturally alkaline diet, consisting of fresh, live foods that we could either pull from the ground or pick from a tree. The word "alkaline" is a key one here because alkaline foods turn to an alkaline ash in the blood and are naturally compatible with our bodies. Alkaline foods cleanse our bodies and provide us with vital energy.

It was easy for our ancestors, all their food was readily available to eat. It was all around them. They didn't have to search for it. They didn't have to hunt. They didn't need to cook it, or even preserve and store it. Every day They woke up and there it was, growing from the soil or hanging from the trees.

We ate with the seasons and enjoyed a wide variety of fruits, vegetables, seeds, nuts and grains. As a result, we were healthy, lean and virtually free of disease. Obesity wasn't a problem. Every vitamin, mineral, protein, carbohydrate and essential fat we needed was present in the natural raw foods that grew from the ground.

We moved away from natural raw foods and embraced newer versions. So much so that we now seem to have forgotten that the correct fuel for our bodies is still the food of the land.

Sadly, for most people, fresh raw food now makes up only a small portion of their diet, if at all. And therein the problem lies. When we eat natural foods, we have all the enzymes we need in our bodies to effortlessly convert them into energy, and create health and vitality. Yet we are now so far removed from the foods we used to eat, and our bodies are suffering the consequences.

One of the major problems is that we are constantly being lied to by the food industry. We are brainwashed into accepting that certain foods are healthy without questioning the ingredients or the credibility of the claims. Who says these new modern day foods are healthy? The food companies, that's who! But where does their information come from? What makes them the experts? And are they telling us the truth?

···➤ *ASSUME makes an ASS out of U and ME!*

All you have to do is look at the epidemic of sickness and obesity to see for yourself that something is seriously amiss. And you won't have to look very far.

Literally everybody must know someone who is overweight or sick. Hippocrates said "Let food be your medicine and medicine be your food". Yet it seems food is now man's poison, not his medicine.

Before some bright spark invented the refrigerator, we were preserving, pickling, salting, smoking and canning food, but mostly we had to eat everything fresh or it would simply go off. Now, not only do we keep food longer in the fridge, but it is also highly processed to make it last longer still. We can now keep it for years without even the need for a fridge. Chemicals and additives are loaded into foods and drinks without our consent. Yet they are incompatible with our bodies and are also making us fat. And more besides - Attention Deficit Syndrome and Hyperactivity are just two recently discovered conditions known to be associated with food.

In truth, we are all genetic experiments in the process. If things don't change the long-term effects will be disastrous. We are living in the age of fast food and, logically enough, we are getting fat and sick fast. I can't say it often enough: we are simply not designed to eat processed foods and we are poisoning our bodies every time we do so. This is now the first generation where parents will outlive their children. That's sickening news.

To process a food, the energy has to be taken out of it. This prevents bacteria thriving. However, if it's not good enough for bacteria then why is it good enough for us? Get it straight now: processed foods are dead foods. If you want to live you need to eat fresh, live foods that contain vital nutrients, enzymes and energy. The further away a food is from nature, the worse it is for your body.

⋯➤ *You can LIVE-IT or DIE-T. The choice is yours. LIVE foods give you LIFE!*

Fear for the future

Never before have we had such a high incidence of heart disease, diabetes and cancer. Yet what saddens me most is the incidence of obesity and diabetes type two in children. They are our future, yet I fear for their health and also the effect on their mental well-being of the world we are creating for them.

If you have children, I urge you to take action and start looking carefully at the ingredients in the foods they are eating. As a mother of two young boys, I was shocked when I eventually plucked up the courage to do this. I also felt enormous guilt for the chemicals and additives I had unknowingly allowed my children to consume. For example, I had always encouraged them to drink sugar-free drinks, thinking this was the best choice. Wrong! It was the worst possible choice, but I had been brainwashed.

As you can imagine, my new-found concerns created quite a stir at home. In fact, I have been ridiculed by friends and family alike for being fanatical. Yet if I can't be fanatical about my children's health, then what can I be? If you're fussy about the fuel you put in your car, are you called a fanatic or a car freak? Of course not.If your child developed a disease due to bad diet you would be expected to be fanatical about finding a cure. However, I'm interested in prevention not cure, so call me fanatical if you choose.

I look it at like this: I have an obligation to protect my children from the lies and deceit blatantly being sold by the food industry. The very least I can do for them while they are growing up is try to influence them to make healthy food choices. After all, their lives depend on it.

Do you care more about putting the right petrol in your car than the right ingredients in your children or grandchildren's food? Unfortunately, this is true for most of the population. I would rather make a stand now and make them aware of it, than wait until they're faced with a serious health crisis such as diabetes or cancer. Too many people wait until a crisis hits before making a change, and I don't want to be one of them. When my kids fly the nest, of course they will find their own way. Yet I feel sure that my influence will have had a positive impact.

As well as my immediate family, I am also blessed with lots of nephews, nieces and godchildren. Yet despite the information I share with family and friends, they still let their children drink sodas that contain the lethal ingredient, aspartame. Perhaps I'm too close to home to be taken seriously, I don't know. Maybe after they read this book they will think again. I certainly hope so.

As I will discuss in detail, additives and chemicals are deliberately being put into our children's foods to make them addicted, to make them fat and to increase the size of their appetite. If they get them hooked now, they've got them for life. Before you say "Surely they wouldn't do that?" just reflect on this crucial fact: the food industry relies on addiction to increase their profits. It also relies on our ignorance and our lack of interest in added ingredients. I know you are questioning these statements, as I used to myself. But I'm afraid it is only too true, and I will give you all the evidence in a later chapter.

Your car or your body?

To go back to the car analogy, the way we eat now is like putting diesel in a car designed to run on unleaded petrol. Our engines, i.e. our bodies, were simply not designed to digest the types of foods we are consuming. Yet, despite warning signs such as the drastically increased incidences of cancer, heart disease, diabetes, fatigue, poor digestion, obesity and many more conditions, we still continue to punish our bodies and sabotage our health. It's madness!

Sadly, most people take more care of their car than they do their own bodies. No matter how long the queue is at the petrol station, no matter how rushed you were, would you consider putting the wrong type of fuel in your car? Of course not. You know full well it would ruin the engine. Well, that is exactly what you are doing when you put processed foods into your engine.

Just think about it for a moment. How many times do you put food into your mouth, oblivious of the ingredients? Yet why do you trust the food manufacturers? Do you know them personally? Do you think they care about your health? Ignoring what's being put in your food is like pulling up to the petrol pump and putting any old stuff in the tank…hey, fuel is fuel, right? Wrong, wrong, wrong! You wouldn't do this in a million years. But I know you eat foods without looking at the ingredients first.

You have to realise that food is not food anymore. At least, the majority of "foods" in the supermarkets aren't. They didn't grow. They were designed for one reason only, to make the food industry rich. And the food industry is very devious. Every year, thousands of food-like substances hit the shelves. I say "food-like" because that's what they are. Low fat, low carb, fortified, processed, low sugar and low calorie; anything but Mother Nature's fuel for the human body.

For the purpose of this book, I want you to imagine your body is a beautiful car. Choose any car you want, as exotic as you like – Ferrari, Lamborghini, Bentley – whatever turns you on. This car is the car of your dreams. In addition, it has to be extremely reliable because it's going to take you all the way on your journey through life. You won't be able to trade it in until you die, so think carefully about your choice.

Your car, like your body, has to run on four elements: fuel, oil, water and air. If just one of these elements were missing, your vehicle would struggle to function and eventually break down. Your body is exactly the same. Without a well-balanced diet, each individual cell and the overall structure begin to break down. The first symptoms are fatigue, weight gain and premature ageing, followed by disease and an early death.

···➤ *We're digging our own graves with our knives and forks*

Nature's early warning system. Death
The very fact you are overweight means your body is not functioning the way it was designed to. Luckily, weight gain is an external symptom that prompts us to make changes. However, most people focus only on losing the weight with no regard for their general state of health; how many internal symptoms are you suffering without knowing? The first sign of a heart attack is usually death!

It was my own struggle with weight that started my quest for perfect health. There are many people who seem to be fit slim and healthy on the outside and then suddenly drop dead. Because they had no external symptoms, they and everyone around them assumed they were healthy. But here's another vital point to grasp.

Health is not merely the absence of disease. If you are one of those people who always feel tired despite sleeping well, it's time to start seriously questioning your state of health. Fatigue is not a normal condition; it's often a symptom of something more serious.

You have to look beyond the symptom to the cause.

In most cases, fatigue can be eliminated totally by eating foods that contain high water content, nutrients, energy and, above all, enzymes. Fatigue is one of Mother Nature's warning signs. To ignore it, or even worse accept it, is suicidal.

Now, I am assuming you are reading this book because you want to lose weight, which is great. As I've said, though, it's not just about losing weight. Losing weight is simply a process which gets you to a place where you feel better about yourself. You also want more energy, greater health and to live a longer life. All reasons why I want you to listen to what I'm about to tell you very carefully. If you want to transform your body, it's some of the most important information you are ever going to learn.

···➤ *In order to change, you have to accept that you need to change.*

Fat, sick and poisoned!

If you think the food manufacturers care about what they put in your food, you are very wrong. And if you think you can trust the government to force them to act appropriately, wrong again. In this world, you have to take responsibility for making sure you know what goes into your own body. You need to know the effect it has on your health and internal organs. Only then can you make an intelligent choice.

To function on all cylinders and to have outstanding health, we must eat the fuel we were designed to eat. Don't panic, however. I'm not asking you to eat like a rabbit, as you will see.

Essentially, the goal of the food companies is to make money. As publicly traded corporations, they are required to increase profits and shareholder value. To this end, their primary objective is to sell more of their products. They simply want to sell more and more food. Indeed, their publicly stated objectives are to get more and more people consuming larger and larger amounts of food.

Manufacturers produce food by using genetic engineering and food processing techniques. They add chemicals, colourings and preservatives that create disease and make you fat.

For example, sweeteners are just one of many chemicals that not only make you sick but also make you put on weight. Yet children's foods are now being loaded with this deadly poison.

Diet foods, low fat foods and sugar free and low sugar drinks are all full of aspartame, which you may know better as NutraSweet and Splenda. You will find a whole chapter on the dangers of this product, which will blow your mind. It's also now accepted that artificial colours lead to hyperactivity and anxiety, especially in children, but when are we going to recognise the link to other, more fatal conditions?

···➤ *If you can't spell it, don't eat it*

A way to ensure that we consume more food is to put addictive chemicals into our food. Aspartame, high fructose corn syrup and sugar are just three of these.

True, trans fats and hydrogenated fats are finally being labeled on the foods we eat, but this isn't because the food industry has suddenly become concerned about our well-being. It's because the destructive effects of these lethal fats are ruining the lives of millions of people.

It's costing the NHS a fortune, but this is great news for the pharmaceutical industry. At last the government is facing facts and beginning to coerce the food industry into correctly labelling their foods.

This won't happen overnight, however, so in the meantime people are still unknowingly consuming who knows what on a daily basis, and the damage escalates.

I think this situation is disgraceful and it angers me greatly. We are indirectly being lied to. We are being made to believe we are eating healthy foods because the foods aren't labeled "Unhealthy". In the early 1900s, any food that was not real had to be labeled "Imitation".

Needless to say, that rule didn't last long; can you imagine if that law still existed? Apart from the peripheral aisles in the supermarkets, almost everything would have to be labeled "Imitation". Now, that would heighten awareness – which is exactly why the rule was quashed. How very, very sad. And what a comment on humanity.

If we can't rely on the food industry or the government to protect us, we have to get wise and take responsibility for our own lives.

Going up in smoke

There is an obvious parallel to all this. For over 50 years, the tobacco companies flagrantly lied to the public and the supreme courts. Under oath, they denied tobacco caused lung cancer and many other fatal diseases. They spent billions bribing and paying off officials. Huge advertising campaigns promoted how cool and trendy smoking was. Youngsters were impressed, bought into the lies and then became addicted. Of course, with millions of people addicted sales increased year on year.

Finally, after many successful lawsuits, the real truth emerged and the tobacco companies were exposed. Yet how many innocent people died as a result of those lies? The wonderful entertainer, Roy Castle, was one of those innocent victims. Despite never smoking a cigarette in his life, he died of a particular kind of lung cancer only found in smokers. In other words, he died of passive smoking.

Roy's death was not in vain, however. It raised the profile of the anti-smoking lobby, and his wife fought tirelessly on its behalf. I believe she had a great influence on the national smoking ban that followed.

It's only a matter of time before we see the same type of lawsuit being filed against the food conglomerates here in the UK, once the effects of the lethal chemicals being added to our foods begin to manifest and are fully researched. I sincerely hope it's never you or a member of your family filing one of those lawsuits. It may take another 50 years, but it will happen, you'll see.

In the meantime, the food industry will carry on working tirelessly to seduce our children. A toy with a happy meal or cereals has always worked wonders. Further on, you'll find a list of the addictive chemicals being added to your everyday foods. You will also learn the detrimental effects they have on your mind and body. None of these ingredients can be found in fresh natural foods.

By now it goes without saying, but I'll say it anyway: avoid processed food whenever you can. In nature, there is usually an antidote within a metre of any poison. The only antidotes to additives are pharmaceutical drugs. Have you ever considered that the food and drug industries might be in cahoots?

During your lifetime you will have many cars and a few different homes, but you will have only one body. The health of that body is a direct reflection of the choices you make every day, simple as that.

Whether you choose to care for your body or neglect it, it's entirely down to you. Many of the conditions and diseases you suffer are caused by your choice of foods. However, the good news is that you can easily rectify them.

It's time now to get your priorities right and start looking after the most precious vehicle you'll ever have, your own wonderful body. If you don't look after your body you will have nowhere to live.

Animal magic

In the wild there are no overweight animals. Nor do they suffer from heart disease, cancer, arthritis or diabetes. Funnily enough there's no depression either. This is because they stay in their natural habitat and continue to eat a natural, raw, live alkalarian diet. They simply weren't intelligent enough to deviate. Lucky them!

With plentiful food sources, animals remain on the whole healthy and well nourished.

To this day, animals are able to fully digest and absorb their food, which in turn converts to energy. It's common to see different size animals in the wild, but you will never find a fat one wobbling around. Hippos and elephants might appear fat, but this is the way nature intended them to be. Even when they are starving they still look fat.

Wild animals eat slowly and simply, eating one food group at a time. Equally significantly, they do not drink while they eat. They drink before and after a meal, but never during it. They instinctively know that drinking water will dilute the digestive juices, rendering digestion inefficient and requiring too much energy.

It's highly significant that the only animals that suffer from "human diseases" are domestic animals – dogs, cats, horses, guinea pigs, etc.

We share our foods with our pets, thinking we are being kind when, in fact, we are punishing them by encouraging them to eat the wrong grade fuel and poisoning their bodies. The result is that vets can earn more than doctors. Animals were simply not designed to eat processed food, and neither were you.

"All truth passes through three stages.
First, it is ridiculed.
Second, it is violently opposed.
Third, it is accepted as being self-evident."
ARTHUR SCHOPENHAUER

ACID: THE BURNING ISSUE

"There is only one disease, the over-acidification of the body."
ROBERT O YOUNG, PHD

CAN I LET YOU INTO A SECRET? WHEN YOU ARE OVER-weight, it is not actually a fat problem at all. It's an acid problem. This is not so much a secret as a scientifically researched fact. Dr. Robert O. Young, author of The pH Miracle, states that fat is created to bind acidity into the body and store it away from its vital organs and delicate systems. To me, this makes perfect sense.

Dr. Young believes – as I do, from my own experience – that as you consume extra acid the body goes into self-preservation mode. In order to protect itself, it produces more fat cells. These act like a sponge and soak up the excess acid. The more acid you consume, the more fat cells you need to produce. This is why whenever I see a fat person, I know it's a symptom of an acidic lifestyle.

This means your fat could be saving your life and that without it you'd be dead.

Not understanding that an acid diet means fat development explains why so many people yo-yo back and forth on one diet after another. Diet foods are highly acidic and so just perpetuate the problem. All foods convert to an ash in the blood stream, whether acid, alkaline or neutral.

Yet diet and other processed foods create acid ash that can compromise your health.

When you understand the real purpose of fat and how and why it is developed, you can appreciate how changing the way you live, eat and think can help you.

And when you no longer have to experience this fat storing reaction, you can lose weight, change your body and your health without dieting.

Yippee!

Disease means dis-ease

Only 40 years ago, people were slim in Great Britain; the Americans envied us. Processed foods had not reared their ugly heads and the majority of the foods we consumed were fresh and prepared daily. Heart disease and cancer were less common, while people ate mostly to satisfy hunger and refuel their bodies. There were no addictive chemicals added to our food, and consequently obesity was much rarer..

Today, the evidence is very clear. Despite great leaps in medical research, and the many new treatments and drugs available, as a nation we are getting fatter and fatter and sicker and sicker. There are over 25,000 diets on the market; we are bombarded with diet and low fat foods and yet the epidemic is getting progressively worse every day. Just go and stand in your "common sense corner" for a minute.

Do you agree that something just doesn't add up here? Our ancestors were fit and healthy and suffered far less from the killer diseases around today, those sometimes referred to as "diseases of affluence".

Amazingly, man has survived for thousands of years without the need for calorie counting or nutritionists.

However did we do it? It wasn't so long ago that we British used to look at our American cousins in horror as we witnessed the growing epidemic of obese children and adults. Now we too are becoming a fat, sick nation. What really scares me is the fact that we appear to be simply accepting it.

I suggested earlier that you imagine yourself waking up one morning to find your body bloated and a couple of stones heavier than the night before.

How tired and depressed you'd feel, with your clothes tight and your self-esteem and confidence low. As I said, you do have a disease and it's called being overweight. The very word disease means "*dis-ease*"; i.e. your body is out of ease and uncomfortable with itself. Do not for one moment try to convince yourself that you or your body are at ease being overweight. Being overweight is a burden to your physical body and your emotional well-being. Perfect weight means your body is *at-ease*.

Cooking up trouble

How did all this happen to us, the most intelligent race on the planet? Simply through the introduction of cooked, processed food – acids – that clog the body and slow down its natural rhythms. The main culprit is the consumption of dead, cooked foods that lack enzymes and energy. Enzymes are the life force in food and vital for digestion and providing our cells with energy.

When you consume a diet lacking in enzymes on a regular basis, vital energy conserved for other bodily functions such as burning calories and fat is called upon for digestion. Consequently, these functions are compromised and come to a halt.

You can't have failed to notice that most of our processed foods, fast foods and eating habits are influenced by the USA. Whatever goes on in America usually filters through to Britain. With a McDonald's, Starbucks, Subway and KFC on almost every block, America quickly became the fattest nation on earth. And now we Brits are the second fattest. That's right, we are the second most obese nation in the world, and our biggest killers are the same as those in America.

For good measure, we are also the most constipated nation in Europe. Colon cancer is our second biggest killing cancer. All that cooked food we have been eating is now showing up in various cancers and other major illnesses.

In truth, we don't really know why we started cooking food or killing animals to eat. Maybe it was after the ice age, when natural plantations of food were scarce. Maybe it was at the same time as man discovered fire and he used cooking as a way of preserving.

We do know that fire kills all living things and that preserving became popular when sailors went to sea for a long time. However, they returned with a whole host of conditions, scurvy being just one of them.

When you consume an acidic diet, which is predominantly processed – cooked, dead food lacking in enzymes – your body literally disintegrates. Think about how you tenderise meat. You add acid, which slowly causes the meat to break down. Because of the harmful effects of the acid, you struggle to digest the food which is then stored as toxins and fat – and your body protests.

In a way, fat is your body's way of protesting, so is disease and dis-ease. You literally start to rot from the inside out. You get tired, you get weak and you become ill. Fat is the symptom and acid is the cause. In order to lose weight, you need to address the acid problem by eliminating it from your diet and changing your thoughts. Focusing on the symptom simply isn't enough. Imagine pulling up the weeds in your garden and expecting them not to grow back again. Any gardener would tell you that if you want permanent results you must treat the root cause. To conquer your weight issue, you need to address the cause and eliminate it permanently from your life.

So, how do you eliminate acid from your diet? Simple. You eat more fresh, raw, live foods. You eat more enzymes. You choose nourishing thoughts. All of which are alkalising. Finally, you work with the natural rhythms of your body and not against them.

Death begins in the colon

Often overlooked, an important contributory factor to being overweight is a clogged colon. If your colon is clogged, then so is your body. As I've said before, the process of digestion is the most energetic of all bodily functions.

All other functions will be compromised to create enough energy to digest food. If the colon is clogged, there is tremendous strain on the body and your energy levels will drop dramatically.

Do you have any of the following symptoms:

- **Slow metabolic rate?**
- **Weight gain?**
- **Fatigue?**
- **Bloating?**
- **Flatulence?**
- **Dark circles under the eyes?**
- **Protruding stomach?**
- **Bad breath?**

These are just some of the symptoms associated with a blocked colon. Many of the foods you have been eating, in particular animal flesh, are not suitable for human digestion and therefore get stuck in the large intestine. I should know; I have been a colonic therapist for 13 years. During that time I have treated many patients who were recovering from bowel cancer, and all of them, without a single exception, were advised to avoid eating animal flesh.

It's not hard to see why. There is more detail on this in a later chapter, but I'll summarise the key point now: the length of the human digestive tract is approximately 28 feet. In carnivores it's only four feet. When a lion kills and eats his prey he sleeps for 20 hours. His body is designed to process and digest meat. Yours isn't. A lion produces five times more hydrochloric acid than humans, the acid that breaks down meat. This is the reason why we feel so tired when we eat a meal containing animal flesh. The time it takes to move meat through our body can be as much as 72 hours. During this process your calorie burning power will be switched off, your metabolic rate will drop and your energy level will be extremely low. How do you feel after your Full English breakfast or Sunday roast? This is the reason your poo is so smelly, the animal has been putrefying in your warm body for days.

Unfortunately, it's not just rotting meat that causes this problem. Processed foods have the same negative impact. Because these foods are not "real" and have very low water content, the body cannot utilise them and has difficulty digesting them. Any food not utilised for fuel and tissue repair is stored as toxins and fat.

⋯➤ *What you don't eliminate, you re-circulate.*

Don't cut the "crap"!

One dump or two? If you have less than two bowel movements a day, you probably have a clogged colon. The ideal is three times a day. If you know anyone who's fortunate enough to go three times a day, the chances are they're very slim and healthy.

Lack of water, fibre and digestive enzymes, together with not enough walking and exercising are other contributory factors to the colon becoming clogged. Prescription and non-prescription drugs and excessive caffeine are also to blame. In addition, the times at which you eat particular food types can hinder digestion, as can the way you combine different foods. In autopsies, medical doctors have found as much as 30lbs of undigested fecal matter in people's colons. Yes, 30lbs! If you seriously want to lose weight, you simply must clean up your colon first. From this, everything else will clean up too.

I like to call the colon the "first brain". It's where you feel your feelings first. You must have heard the saying "gut feeling". If you feel excited, nervous, concerned, happy or sad, where do you feel it? Yes, that's right, it's in your gut, not your head. When you clean up your colon, your energy and intuition come back to life.

Colonics are an essential part of my own monthly maintenance. I can't imagine life without them. Indeed, before you do anything else, I recommend you seriously consider a course of colonic hydrotherapy. If you don't want to take that option, there are some wonderful colon cleanses around – for more info look on my website.

Innercleanse is a revolutionary system that enables you to experience the cleansing benefits of colonic whilst still maintaining your privacy and dignity. It's surprisingly comfortable and there's no discomfort or embarrassment whatsoever.

Until you cleanse your colon, your digestion and metabolic rate will remain slow and you will continue to crave foods and have a large appetite. This is because your body is not absorbing sufficient nutrients. To go back to our analogy, think of your colonic as servicing your car. You wouldn't dream of running your car for years without servicing, would you? Well, then! Cleansing the colon is absolutely vital for good health and weight loss.

And in the meantime take a good peep at your poop! A healthy poop should be pale brown, fully formed and float, so check it out. Rectal bleeding must never be ignored, and if you have any bleeding contact your doctor immediately. Urine should be clear or straw coloured. The colour of your urine and poops are your body's way of telling you what's going on inside. It's estimated that up to 10% of colon cancers could be prevented if the symptoms had been spotted earlier.

■ TAKE THE P...

Check out your urine. If it's:

> **Dark yellow – you're dehydrated**
> **Straw coloured – you're fine**
> **Clear – you're fine too**

It's all in the mind

Negative thoughts such as guilt, failure, frustration, secret eating, bingeing, self-criticism, self-loathing and depression also flood the body with acids. Indeed, the stress of being overweight and on a constant diet is a major factor for the production of acid in the blood. Simply changing what you eat is not enough. For optimum health and a slender body you need to change your thoughts too.

Many people tell me that their weight gain is a genetic tendency. Their parents and grandparents were fat, they say. This may indeed be the case, but with the precious knowledge you're learning, you can make the necessary adjustments to your food intake and lifestyle and stop modelling your body on theirs. It's also very important that you stop believing you'll end up looking like them. Trust me, your beliefs are very powerful and can have unbelievable consequences.

The hoodoo of voodoo

There are still parts of the world where tribal witch doctors practise voodoo and are believed to have magical powers. When someone commits a crime, he is brought before the witch doctor for punishment. The witch doctor shakes a bone and casts a death curse on him, while the other villagers surround him and do the same. The unfortunate criminal is told he is going to die and is then sent off into the bush to do just that. Because his belief is so strong, within 48 hours he is in a coma and within four days he is dead.

This is how powerful beliefs can be. Now, if you were on holiday and were unlucky enough to stumble across a witch doctor and he put the same curse on you, it might unnerve and worry you, but it wouldn't kill you. Why? Because you wouldn't believe it, that's why.

The moral is, you should never underestimate the power of your mind. Every thought you have is transmitted to every cell in your body. This is why hypochondriacs are always ill. They believe they are ill, simple as that. They often have all the symptoms, but the medical diagnosis is inconclusive.

The placebo effect is a classic example of how powerful our thoughts are. If a patient is led to believe medication will cure him and doesn't know he has been given a placebo drug, he can show great improvements in even the most serious illnesses.

···➤ Genetics are the bullet; lifestyle is the trigger

If you want to be slim and healthy, it's all about changing your beliefs and lifestyle. In my opinion, genetics may be the bullet, but lifestyle is the trigger!

Let me share something with you. I have heart disease and cancer on both sides of my family. I consider myself fortunate to know this as it gives me the foresight to make sure the foods I eat and my lifestyle do not contribute to either of these diseases. Stress and diet are two of the biggest contributory factors in heart disease and cancer. When someone has a heart attack, the main recommendation from their consultant is to remove stress from their everyday life. The consultant also advises them to cut down on processed fatty foods, remove saturated fat from their diet and exercise more.

Many people quit their jobs, change careers or leave relationships to accomplish these tasks. After suffering a near death experience, it's amazing what lengths people will go to preserve their bodies. Health suddenly becomes a number one priority and work becomes secondary. Yet health should always be your number one priority because without it you have nothing. It's the nucleus of a happy and fulfilling life. What a pity most of us don't have the foresight to make the changes before a health crisis. Prevention is the absolute cure.

Cancer patients are given the same advice as heart attack victims, with the emphasis on strengthening the immune system by eating nutritionally dense, live foods. Many also remove meat and dairy products from their diet upon diagnosis, as both have been proven to be aggravators. Again, however, most people wait until they fall prey to the disease before making changes. Many others never get the chance and die. Why wait until you are having chemotherapy or are on a life support machine, and suddenly have a moment of realisation through sheer fear?

One that almost got away

Mike, one of my clients, finally decided to call me as he was in the ambulance on his way to Accident and Emergency. (To clarify, he didn't actually call me from the ambulance, but that was where he made the decision to.) He had suffered a massive heart attack. We had spoken several times on the telephone the year before, and he was deliberating as to whether or not he could justify the cost of coming to see me. He had been resistant to all my suggestions, saying he didn't want to

■ HOW ACID ARE YOU?

Do you have any of these symptoms:

- ⌐ EXCESS WEIGHT
- ⌐ LOW ENERGY
- ⌐ POOR DIGESTION
- ⌐ PREMATURE AGEING
- ⌐ FLUID RETENTION
- ⌐ CRAVINGS
- ⌐ DISEASE
- ⌐ ACHES & PAINS
- ⌐ FOGGY THINKING
- ⌐ AFTERNOON "SLUMPS"
- ⌐ MEMORY LOSS
- ⌐ BAD BREATH, DESPITE CLEANING TEETH AND USING MOUTHWASH
- ⌐ ACID REFLUX – HEARTBURN
- ⌐ HEADACHES AND MIGRAINES

0-5? *Well done, but make sure follow my guidelines.*
6-10? *Oh dear! Take immediate action.*
More than 10? *You're drowning in acid. Seek medical help right away.*

feel deprived of the things he liked the most. He lived in a constant state of stress, was overweight and overworked and relied on false stimulants such as 10 cups of coffee a day to keep him going.

In our most recent conversation, I had told him straight: "Mike, if you don't make a change you're heading for a heart attack, I just know it." Sadly, I was right. It wasn't a coincidence but a well educated guess. The frustrating thing was that, despite having prescribed him anti-depressants, his doctor had never suggested any diet or lifestyle changes. You can't treat the human body with such neglect and abuse and expect it to keep functioning. The guy had been sabotaging his life. Mike told me his whole life flashed before him in that ambulance and he realised that the way he was eating and living was depriving him of the very thing he loved the most, life itself!

As soon as he was discharged from hospital, Mike came to see me. I'm pleased to report that he has since lost three stone and has completed his first half marathon. He is a picture of health and enjoying his life to the full. Lucky him, though, for being blessed with a second chance. Oh, I almost forgot, no more anti-depressants for Mike either.

Please, don't you wait until disease sets in before you change. A hospital bed is definitely not the best place to start.

As a child, you may have been told what to eat and where to go, but you are an adult now and you call the shots, nobody else. You have to start taking responsibility for your body and your lifestyle. The state of your body and your health are down to the choices you have made in the past. Today is simply the future you created yesterday. If you want a better life, better body, better health and better job, you need to start making better choices; it's as simple as that.

···➤ *A hospital's job is disease care. Accident and Emergency's is crisis care. Yours is health care.*

Let's get started!

Your first step is to cleanse your blood of all that poisonous acid that's been floating around, perpetuating your weight problem and creating a firm foundation for disease and excess fat. The more acid in your blood stream, the more the body produces fat cells to prevent that acid marinating your organs. Don't forget this fact, it's very important if you want to win the battle of the bulge.

It may help to remember this fish tank metaphor: if your

fish was sick, would you take it to the vet or would you change the water first? If you know your fish, you'd change the water first – and that's exactly what you need to do with your body. Your body is 70-80% water. The water bathes every cell, and those cells are the building blocks for your life. First, let's determine how acidic you think you are.

···➤ *The number one "over the counter" drug in the USA is antacids.*

Antacids were originally designed to counteract the effects of an acidic meal. Now people don't wait for the indigestion, they pop one before they eat the acid…madness!

How do you remove acid from your diet?

The only way to remove acid from your diet is to change the way you think and eat. As we've discussed, negative thoughts, inward thinking and stress create a highly acidic environment. So do prescription drugs, recreational drugs, alcohol and smoking. However the most common cause of over-acidification is the consumption of highly acidic foods. Unfortunately, most people are now consuming a highly acidic diet without even realising. For example, coffee, artificial sweeteners and sodas are some of the most acidic substances you can put in your body. And don't pat yourself on the back if you've switched to decaf – that's just as bad. Anything acid rots your body, simple as that.

You only have to look at the face of an alcoholic and see the way the acid marinates the organs, from the liver to the puffy face with broken veins and the tender red nose. Alcohol is a fast route to ageing.

The foods you eat make their way into your organs and every cell in your body. So, every time you put crap in your body, you yourself are becoming more crap. To get rid of the acid, you must start by cutting out acid foods and incorporating more alkaline foods to neutralise the acid. Then make a real conscious effort to change your way of thinking. This way you'll begin to alkalise and gradually rebalance your body. And remember, positive thoughts create positive feelings and emotions and enhance the immune system. Negative thoughts create negative feelings, suppress the immune system and create depression, disease and weight gain. It's your choice.

···➤ *Every thought you think has a direct effect on your physiology.*

WANT TO KNOW THE REAL REASON YOU'RE FAT?

OF COURSE YOU DO. SO READ ON.

Dieting can address what you eat. Psychotherapy may examine why you eat. But a good nutritional programme encompasses mind and body. To be slender and healthy, you need to nourish both. Most importantly, you must find the reason why you are overweight. As I always tell my clients, your weight is just a symptom of being out of balance. The excess fat that surrounds your skeleton is the symptom, not the cause. Treating the symptom is never the answer. That's what a diet does – and that's why diets don't work.

When a symptom is evident, you must ask what the cause of it is. Ask, "How did I get to this place?" When you find the cause, you must investigate the cause of the cause, until you get to the root. When you finally address this, all the symptoms vanish.

Every single person who suffers with excess weight suffers from a low metabolic rate. In order to burn off your excess weight, you need to reset your metabolic rate and bring it back to normal. Better still, slightly elevate it. Once your metabolic rate is high, you can eat any kind of food you want without gaining weight. You will burn it naturally as fuel and no longer convert it to fat. Now we're talking.

···➤ *On average we eat around 70 tons of food in our lifetime. And 75% of our energy is used to digest it!*

Get the balance right

Quite simply, if you're overweight you are out of balance. What this means is that your body is not functioning the way it was designed to, and the consequences are that you are not digesting your food and assimilating it as energy. Apart from anything else, this is such a waste. After all, in your lifetime, you will eat around 70 tons of food, or roughly one ton every year.

For the body to make healthy cells, this food has to be digested and converted into energy or eliminated as waste. In many cases, however, the elimination process is not working correctly. This leads to low body metabolism, abnormally high food cravings, the desire to eat when not hungry, plus, of course, the storage of excess fat. If you ignore these symptoms or, worse still, accept them as normal, dis-ease sets in and you are bound for a lifetime of suffering.

Also, food not converted to energy is readily converted to fat and toxins. A build-up of toxins has a disastrous effect on the body and may lead in some cases to premature death. What you don't eliminate you will re-circulate. Basically, it gets stuck in transit and re-absorbed into the body and organs, one of the most important of which is the liver.

When digestion is sluggish, many of the symptoms shown are present. They also occur when your diet is lacking enzymes (only found in raw food), the life force of food. Do any of the symptoms described in the panel relate to you? If so, how can you make sure you digest and eliminate properly? Simple. You eat a diet rich in enzymes, and learn to listen to your body. Add a raw salad to every meal. Timing is also critical, so make sure you read below now.

Hard facts to digest
Do you suffer from:

> - **Weight gain leading to obesity**
> - **Bloating and flatulence**
> - **Foul smelling feces (rotting animal flesh)**
> - **Slow or irregular bowel movements**
> - **Lack of energy and fatigue**
> - **Water retention**
> - **Headaches and migraines**

> Acne, spots, dry skin, dull hair and brittle nails
> Bad breath
> Lack of concentration, foggy thinking
> Depression and moodiness
> Cravings for sweet and savoury foods, even when you've just eaten
> Lack of satisfaction
> Obsessive relationship with foods
> Insomnia or restless sleep

How well do you know your body?

Did you know there are only certain designated slots in the day when your body can actually digest the food you eat? The rest of the time it is assimilating and eliminating. Properly digested food cannot be stored as fat, so it's very important you understand how digestion works and how you can influence it in your favour.

If you eat when your body is resting, the food will be stored as toxins and fat. Not exactly rocket science is it? To go back to our analogy, would you dream of filling your car with fuel while you were still driving? Thought not. Yet that's exactly what you are trying to do when you eat at the wrong times. Putting food in your body when it isn't ready to digest it is crazy and a waste of energy. Your body has three natural digestive cycles and you need to know the mechanics to be able to synchronise your eating pattern. This "golden nugget" is going to be extremely helpful, so I ask you to keep it in the forefront of your mind if you're at all serious. If you honour your body, it will honour you.

Digestion starts in the brain

That's right. Digestion begins in the brain, not in the mouth. The second you start thinking about the food you are going to eat, the hypothalamus gland immediately sends a message to the stomach. Digestive juices and hydrochloric acid are sent in preparation to break down the food.

Of course, everybody thinks about food sometimes, but doing it all day is a typical dieters' syndrome. It only serves to make you hungry. Depriving yourself and then dreaming about the foods on your wish list creates constant hunger, which in turn encourages you to eat when your body does not need food.

Let's look at an example. In the morning, you decide you're going to have a piece of chocolate in the evening. That very thought sends a message to the pancreas to release insulin to break down the anticipated sugar. Yet if the sugar doesn't come, your body will go into fat storage mode to absorb all that excess insulin floating around. The chances are you would crave sugar all day and then pig out in the evening. It's literally true when you say things like, "I'm going to put on pounds when I eat that slice of gateau!" So be careful of what you say. Your body is responsive to every single thought you have.

It's said that we have over 75,000 thoughts every single day, and 60,000 are the same ones we had the day before. If your predominant thoughts are negative and focused on being fat, that's what you get more of the next day. I'll remind you again: what we think all day we become. So, again, watch what you think about.

How your digestion works

1. Food enters your mouth.
2. You should chew it slowly. 30-32 times is good, once for every tooth. Your mouth is your blender. Food needs to be broken down to liquid form, as you don't possess cutting blades in your stomach.
3. It mixes with saliva containing the enzyme amylase to break down starches. If you gulp down your food and don't chew mechanically, this stage of digestion is skipped and the rest of the process is compromised.
4. The food is swallowed and processed through the digestive tract.
5. Gastric juices, hydrochloric acid and enzymes in the stomach break down the food to aid absorption

■ HOW LONG IS IT IN YOUR STOMACH?

	MINUTES	HOURS
WATER	0-10	
JUICE FRESHLY SQUEEZED	15-20	
JUICE PASTEURISED		2-3
FRUIT FRESH	30-60	
FRUIT DRIED		1-3
MELONS	30-45	
MOST VEGETABLES FRESH		1-2
TINNED VEGETABLES		2-4
POTATOES		2-3
SALAD	30	
DENSE VEGETABLE PROTEIN		2-3
COOKED MEAT AND FISH		4-6
SHELLFISH		6-8
BREAD		6-8
RICE		4-6
PASTA		6-7

6. It moves to the small intestine. Vitamins, minerals, proteins, complex carbohydrates and fats are sent to different parts of the body for nourishment.
Cells are manufactured from this stage. This stage is natural juicing.

7. Waste and insoluble fibre is passed into the colon ready for elimination. If waste is not eliminated it is re-circulated into the body via the liver. This malfunction compromises health at all cellular levels and creates disease.

⋯➤ *Chew your juice and juice your food!*

Slowly does it

I repeat, chew your food 32 times for proper digestion – once for every tooth. This change alone will accelerate your fat burning and calorie burning capacity. Practise this today and you will be surprised how good your food tastes and how quickly you feel satisfied. At first it may feel strange, and you may feel like you are chewing in "slow motion". Stick with it. To practise slow eating, try this technique. Don't put anything on your fork until you have completely swallowed the previous mouthful. Better still, use chopsticks!

On the whole, slow eaters are slim and fast eaters are fat. As the saying goes, fast is fat, slow is slim. Say it as a mantra when you eat. As soon as you feel satisfied, stop eating. This is your body's ingenious signal to tell you your fuel tank is full.

■ 10 STEPS TO CREATING A SLENDER, HEALTHY BODY

STEP	
1	CHOOSE POSITIVE HEALTHY THOUGHTS THAT NOURISH YOUR MIND. USE POSITIVE AFFIRMATIONS DAILY.
2	ELIMINATE POISONS THAT PUNISH YOUR BODY.
3	PROPERLY COMBINE YOUR FOODS – MORE ON THIS SOON.
4	DRINK MORE WATER. DRINK HALF YOUR BODY WEIGHT IN OUNCES EVERY DAY.
5	EAT WHEN YOU ARE RELAXED, AND ENJOY EVERY MOUTHFUL.
6	EAT SMALLER PORTIONS.
7	INCREASE YOUR OXYGEN LEVELS.
8	CLEAN YOUR COLON WITH REGULAR COLONICS.
9	LEARN TO REDUCE STRESS.
10	GET MOVING! FIND AN EXERCISE YOU LOVE AND EXERCISE A MINIMUM OF FIVE TIMES A WEEK.

Satisfied says "enough" and full says "it's time to store fat".

Just a few weeks of doing this will transform your body and reduce your appetite massively. The stomach is a very flexible organ that expands and shrinks very quickly. When you overeat for a few consecutive days, you will notice your appetite increases. Conversely, when you eat small portions of nutritionally dense foods, you will notice your appetite shrinks quickly too. And remember, it's a proven fact that light eaters live longer.

Keep your foods simple

⋯➤ *Simple foods are simply digested.*

From this moment onwards, your most important goal is to transport food through your body as quickly as possible. This puts the least strain on your energy requirements and stops undigested foods being stored as fat. Remember, the process of digestion is the most taxing of all bodily functions and requires the most energy – over 75%. Your reserved energy can then be used to heal and replenish cells, and burn calories and fat. Yes, burning fat. That's what you want, right?

On the other hand, putting dense, cooked foods through the digestive system clogs the body and, over time, puts enormous strain on your immune system due to the lack of enzymes. The process of burning fat requires energy, and if you don't have enough energy because the foods you eat are cooked and lifeless, weight loss will be an uphill struggle your whole life long.

Take a look at the transit times on the table opposite. These are the length of time it takes for various food groups to leave your stomach. From then, there's another transit time before food reaches the anus and is eliminated. Raw fruit only takes six hours, raw vegetables 15 hours, while bread takes as long as 24 hours or one day. In the case of animal flesh, it's anything up to 72 hours – three whole days.

Alcohol, aspirin and caffeine penetrate the stomach walls

very quickly, which is why we feel an instant "hit". Alcohol and caffeine are known as "protoplasmic poisons", which mean as soon as they hit a cell they destroy it. Your aim should be to not eat anything until your stomach is empty, so you can get your food through your body as quickly as possible. Understanding transit times is like knowing the quickest route for your car journey. In other words, vital.

Wear your body

It is said that there are over 700 trillion cells in the body, and every single day of your life over 300 billion die off. These 300 billion have to be replaced. And do you know what the replacement cells are made from? Yep, the food you are eating.

There are no truer words spoken than, "You are what you eat". Knowing this makes it even more important that you choose the quality of your foods with great care. Your body is a magnificent machine and ever-changing. It's like a stream, in that you can never step in the same spot twice. If you step in a stream and step out, then try to get back to the same place, you can't because the old water has gone and new water is flowing in. The same applies to the human body. It is ever altering, ever-growing. Each one of those 700 trillion cells is constantly renewing itself, without you consciously being aware. In a sense, you wear your body like a loose garment. Your bones, skin and organs change at the blink of an eye. For example, did you know you get:

> ➤ A new skeletal system every three months
> ➤ A new liver every 10 weeks
> ➤ A new stomach lining every six weeks

So your health and your body weight really do depend on yesterday's meal. Remember, a healthy body will find its own perfect weight, an unhealthy body will hold on to fat as a protection mechanism. Without food, you cannot make new cells and you will wither and die. And no one can argue with that ultimate fact of life.

DITCH
THE
DOUBLE ACT

Food combining makes all the difference

Here's another golden nugget. To ensure you digest key nutrients properly, you simply must know how to effectively combine your foods. If you do this, your digestive organs will continue to work as intended and your food can be easily broken down. You'll also expend less energy in digesting, which will enable you to absorb more nutrients to create new energy and burn fat. However, if you don't combine foods properly, you'll put your body through a lot of unnecessary strain as you digest. It's not exactly the end of the world, you will still digest, but you'll also be wasting vital energy that could be used to burn fat instead. Wrongly combining foods will definitely slow down weight loss and tire you out.

While you're digesting that fact, consider this: have you ever seen an animal eat more than one food group at a time? No. Nor will you see a wild animal overweight, constipated or suffering from food allergies. Even domesticated animals eat and then drink, knowing not to dilute their digestive juices.

As I keep on saying...Throughout your lifetime, 75% of all the energy you expend will be used to break down that 70 tons of food you'll eat. So the idea here is to conserve as much energy as possible by eating foods that require minimal digestion, and learn to combine them properly. Just to remind you again, this process provides maximum energy to burn surplus fat. The body cannot and will not burn fat if it has to reserve energy for digestion. The less energy you need to digest, the more fat you burn, got it?

If you ignore this natural rule, you will feel constantly tired and fatigued. Toxins will accumulate and disease may well seize an opportunity.

The body's response to low energy is to revert to preservation mode, and guess what that means for you? Yes, good old fat storage, the very thing you are working so hard against. The only place you can store surplus energy is the fat cells, and the only way to slow down your energy expenditure is to slow down you too. Your metabolic rate, calorie and fuel burning are all forced to slow down with you. Ever felt tired after a cooked breakfast, Christmas dinner or a Sunday roast meal? Well now you know why.

It's also no coincidence that children are often ill after Halloween, or that there are outbreaks of colds and flu at New Year. A cold, fever or flu is the body's natural way of cleansing itself. I call it a "self-cleanse". The very worst thing that you can do is to bung it up with a decongestant. A symptom such as a headache, ache or pain is a protest, so you must listen to your body. What goes in must come out. Fluids allow the body's natural healing process to take place, as they transport the toxins out in urine and sweat.

As I've said, to accelerate weight loss and generate energy and vitality, your aim is to transport foods quickly and efficiently through your body. Properly digested food cannot be stored as fat.

Look at a squirrel that eats nuts all day, is he fat? No; he eats a shed load of nuts and still seems to have the energy to climb trees and walls at Mach 2. The reason is the squirrel, like all other wild species, eats one food group at a time. He doesn't drink while he eats, and what's even more interesting is that even in the depths of winter he stops when he's satisfied. So next time someone tells you nuts are fattening, say like hell they are. Nuts, like fruit, avocados and many other foods, are not fattening provided you know how and when to eat them.

In truth, if you only choose three steps to follow from this book, food combining would be the third most important. Eating fruit and live foods would be the first and second. And if you're wondering what you'll ever do with all this surplus energy you'll amass, first you can burn that fat from your butt, and second you can start enjoying life. Not a bad reward, is it?

You've had your chips

Now I'm going to go into a bit more detail. I'll make this as simple as possible because you did not come here for a biology lesson. However, if you want a deeper understanding of the science behind food combining I suggest you read *Food Combining Made Easy* by Herbert Shelton.

Right, let's go. There are three main food groups - carbohydrates, fats and proteins. The enzyme required to break down starches and carbohydrates is an alkaline called amylase, and the one needed to break down protein is an acid called pepsin. Now, do you remember that experiment you did at school? If you mix vinegar – acid – with baking soda – alkaline – they neutralise each other and the liquid expands and overflows out of the container within seconds. Well, this is exactly what happens when you eat carbs and proteins together. It's the most common reason for bloating and gas.

How simple was that explanation? I hope you now understand the negative impact of incorrect food combining. In addition to the bloating and gas, which is extremely uncomfortable and embarrassing for some, there is a more serious issue to consider here. If your digestive enzymes are neutralising each other, it means your food is difficult to digest. And do you remember what I told you about undigested foods? That's right, they're stored as toxins and fat.

This will not pose a massive problem if you occasionally eat this way, but doing it constantly will have a significant impact on both your health and your girth. The British and American diets are the worst for combining the wrong food groups at one meal. In fact, almost everything we eat is a combination of the two: fish and chips; chicken and rice; meat and potatoes. You name it,we combine it. We're also both nations of sandwich lovers, and put practically anything and everything on bread and toast.

Bacon sandwich was it, madam?

··· ➤ *Always have a live salad or veg as a substitute for your carbohydrate choice.*

Confused? Good! It means you're about to learn something
I want to remind you that health is not simply the absence of disease. You can't see anything on the outside until it's already developed or grown on the inside. A cancer tumour doesn't show up until it's protruding. Stomach cancer doesn't show until the pain sets in. Heart disease and colon cancer are progressive illnesses that take years to develop. They never happen overnight. They are manifesting while we go about our daily lives, blissfully unaware until we notice a symptom. The problem is, too many people ignore the symptom. We all know people who were absolutely fit and healthy until they found a lump, then overnight are diagnosed with cancer. Many people suffer with fatigue and weight gain, accepting it as normal, only to be told it's diabetes. In that very moment, their whole lives change. But the reality is, it didn't really change overnight. It probably took years, and could have easily been avoided. This was simply the moment they became aware and their fear set in, and their conscious life changed. Sadly, the physical one had already changed.

The majority of diseases known to man are unknowingly self-inflicted, with neglect of the nutritional needs of the body the chief culprit. Now, don't get me wrong. I am not saying this neglect was a conscious choice.

For many people it isn't. Most know no better, have no understanding of how the human body works and, most importantly, what it needs.

Unless you have a particular interest in nutrition, you rely on the information passed down by teachers. Yet who are these teachers? What makes them authorities on the subject? Usually they are your parents, carers, siblings, friends and acquaintances. And who do you think taught them? The media, diet, food and drug industry, of course. Those lovely people who have but one goal – to make money.

These food and drug conglomerates are in bed with each other and have no concern about the state of your health. Most people are on a "High Fact" diet. There are so many controversial facts, so many diets and so much confusion out there, it's mind blowing. So people hear what they want to hear, dismiss what they don't like and adapt what they do like. And this is exactly how eating habits and advice are passed on. The source of the information comes via constant bombardment and brainwashing by the media.

Kevin Trudales' fascinating book *Natural Cures They Didn't Want You To Know*, reveals the great lengths the conglomerates go to lie and conceal the truth about the harmful effects of the foods we're eating. Did you know there have been cures found for cancer? No, didn't think you knew, not many people do. Can you imagine how much money would be lost if a cure for cancer was revealed? If you want to know more about the corruption of the pharmaceutical industry, read Kevin's book, it's a real eye opener.

···➤ *There's only one cure for cancer available to you right now: it's called prevention.*

If you bypass the crap you're being fed by the media and the food companies, and revert back to Mothers Nature's wisdom, you'll see food combining has always been in existence and is the easiest way for the body to digest food efficiently.

Now, let's look at what else is making you fat.

···➤ *If you're still tired after seven to eight hours sleep, something is wrong.*

STRESS MAKES YOU FAT TOO

ANOTHER GAME: SPELL "STRESSED" BACKWARDS. THAT'S right, "desserts". Funny, isn't it? And every time your body feels and reacts to stress, you can literally put on as much weight as if you'd eaten a dessert. Now, that is food for thought.

Ironically, stress is one of the single biggest contributors to both malnutrition and weight gain. You could be eating the healthiest food in the universe, but if you are eating with stress you won't receive the metabolic value from the meal and your body will store it instead of converting it to energy.

Stress is the body's response to any real or imagined threat. Every time you have a stressful thought you release two chemicals called cortisol and adrenaline into your body. Adrenaline is known as the "Fight or Flight" hormone and is released when you experience fear. Cortisol signals your body to store weight as fat and not to build muscle. At the same time as these reactions, blood rushes to your extremities and away from the stomach. Digestion is switched off to enable you to deal with the oncoming danger and save the body vital energy. The type of fat resulting is usually apparent on the abdomen.

Here's an example of how this would have worked when we were cavemen. Let's say you're sitting eating your meal, nice and relaxed. All of a sudden a sabre-toothed tiger comes to the opening of your cave and gets ready to pounce on you. You drop your food with fright. Immediately, your heart starts to race and your blood pressure goes up. You start to shake with fear and your stomach begins to churn. Faced with the threat, your body immediately shuts off digestion and sends blood and energy to your arms and legs so you can run and fight.

Next, adrenaline and cortisol martial extra energy to help you deal with the fear and fight off the tiger. You fight off the tiger and then, phew, you are done! As you begin to relax, digestion is switched back on again. You head back to your cave feeling exhausted and as you walk through the doorway you suddenly feel ravenous. You go back into your cave and sit down to the evening meal you now richly deserve.

Does this scenario sound familiar to you? Are you a caveman? Rather more likely, is your work or lifestyle the tiger? The trouble is, the caveman scenario is how "Fight or Flight" reactions were meant to work: helping us to deal with danger and then switching off when the danger is over. Sadly, the way millions of stressed people live their daily lives is with their "Fight or Flight" switched on the whole time– in a constant state of fear. The physiological response is exactly the same as if the threat were physical and real; the difference is they are experiencing it all day, every single day of their lives. Constant use of the adrenal glands will eventually lead to burnout, and boy, if your adrenal glands burn out you are in big trouble.

Sadly, people experience stress in the form of fear every day. Fear of being stuck in traffic. Fear of being late. Fear of being sacked. Fear of losing somebody. Fear of hurting somebody. Fear of being hurt. Fear of not being good enough. Fear of not getting everything done. Fear of the unknown. Fear of losing money. Fear of missing a phone call. Fear of losing their health. Fear of death. Fear of being overweight. Fear of... and so it goes on and on and on.

Fright is a natural feeling, but fear could be defined as a constant state of fright. If you are constantly living your life under the stress, the body perceives this to be fear and pumps out those harmful, acidic chemicals, adrenaline and cortisol. The more of these chemicals are released, the more fat cells are produced to soak them up.

Have you notice how much older you look after only a few days of stress?

In other words, stress makes you fat and it's incredibly ageing.

To me, stress means you are giving something more significance than it deserves. If you are one of those people who suffer stress, perhaps now is a good time to make some changes in your life. How about taking up meditation or having a holiday? What do you say to changing career? or at least starting to exercise?

There is nothing more stressful than spending your life worrying about what you look like, how much you weigh, why you can't lose weight and what you can't wear. Being overweight is stressful; for most of us it's a negative thought that consumes our everyday life.

Conversely, finding your ideal weight by focusing on health and nutrition is a positive experience that releases the burden of stress. There are enough challenges in life without you having to deal with your weight; let the weight drop and you will feel free, light and empowered.

So, it's clear that under stress you don't digest. People who experience prolonged stress on a daily basis normally store weight around the midriff. The body will store weight around this area even if you don't overeat, so stress alone is enough to cause a long-term weight problem.

The most significant danger of this excess fat is its location around the heart and other major organs. I'm sure you have heard the phrase "stress is a killer". It's absolutely true. Negative thoughts have a disastrous effect on the heart, weakening the muscle and valves and poisoning the surrounding major organs.

Breathe your way through it

There is a simple way to cut the stress response within a minute and go from no to full digestive power. Can you guess what it is? (Clue in the title!) Yes, it's all about breathing.

Every brain state and every emotional state has a corresponding breathing pattern. The breathing pattern of stress is shallow, arrhythmic and infrequent. In contrast, the breathing pattern of relaxation is regular, rhythmic and deep. If you adopt the breathing of a relaxed person, you literally fool your body. It then thinks it is relaxed and turns digestion back on again.

This is why eating at your desk, in the car, standing up or while rushing around causes weight gain. The body thinks it's under stress because you are distracted or buzzing about and immediately shuts down digestion. Of course, the undigested food is usually stored as fat. Secret eating, feelings of guilt or shame also have the ability to shut down digestion.

How interesting is that? Your body needs to be in a state of relaxation before you eat. When you combine oxygen with food you get calorie burn. Yet it doesn't matter what type of food you are eating, if there is not enough oxygen, you're not fully digesting your meal.

Turn on your other half

Nothing steamy, I'm afraid! There are two simple "switches" in your brain. Part of the autonomic nervous system, they're called the sympathetic and parasympathetic nervous systems. The sympathetic nervous system turns on stress and turns off digestion. Conversely, the parasympathetic system turns on the relaxation response that is full, healthy digestive and calorie burning power.

In other words, the same part of your brain that is responsible for turning on stress shuts down digestion and the same part that relaxes you gives you the fullest metabolic force. There's nothing new here, either. This information has been around for 75 years, and it's long been known that the state of relaxation is the optimal state for digestion and relaxation.

No wonder, either, that many European countries take a two hour break every day. They stop work, have a long, leisurely lunch and relax fully before going back to work. The fact that they eat foods such as bread and cheeses and then swill it down with a few glasses of wine doesn't cause a weight problem because they're so relaxed. A power lunch is not normal in these cultures. Pound for pound, the French are the largest consumers of fat in the world and yet are also one of the slimmest of nations. They also pay no attention to food combining, however they eat a raw salad with each meal and combine proteins and starches mainly at midday, giving the body adequate time to digest the foods. The other thing to consider is the quality of their food is fresh and mainly free from preservatives. I suggest if you want to combine carbs and protein, the best time would be at lunch.

So do they have a secret? They sure do: it's called a positive relationship with food. They eat fresh, delicious foods and take the time to prepare them with love. They eat in a relaxed manner, slowly, savoring both the food and the company. They not only nourish their bodies but also their minds. Practically any food can be nourishing, providing you eat it in a nourishing environment, without feelings of guilt or shame.

We Brits, on the other hand, do the opposite.

We rush lunch, skip breakfast, watch TV and eat so fast we can barely taste the food. We sit in clinical environments like offices and cars and even stand up while eating. No longer satisfied with our morning cuppa, we walk round clutching paper cups with something that looks like coffee as if it were the Holy Grail. We constantly graze between meals, as if there's going to be a food shortage. To perpetuate our weight issue even more, we then experience feelings of guilt or deprivation as we swallow.

No wonder we can't digest our food. Remember, negative feelings are feelings of stress. The body reacts by shutting digestion off and flooding you with acid. Have you ever had indigestion or heartburn after rushing your meal? No surprise there. You must realise that food is not the enemy; it's your friend and your medicine. You need to develop a healthy relationship with food if you are to achieve a naturally slim, healthy body. In fact, it's vital you learn to make friends with both the foods you eat and your body, no matter what shape or size it is right now.

Do "do lunch"

A major benefit of eating your largest meal at midday, as the French do, is the position of the sun. Around noon, the sun's energy is at its highest and this helps your digestive power. When the sun is at the max, so is your digestion. For this reason, I would always recommend you try to eat your largest meal at this time.

Eating earlier on in the day also gives your body time to digest your food. The French are so slim partly because by the evening they've fully digested their big meal and feel satisfied, emotionally, physically and nutritionally. There's simply no need to snack when you are satisfied in all these areas.

Equally importantly, "doing lunch" properly gives you the energy you need to get through the day. After all, you probably wouldn't bother filling your car when you get home at night, because it's only going to sit on the drive. So why fill your own tank when you are going to sit on the couch all night? A small evening meal is perfect.

Before some bright spark invented the light bulb, we always used to eat our biggest meal in the middle of the day. Now, because we have light whenever we need it, our days are getting longer. Yet our biological clocks are messed up as a result. Animals eat in the day and so should you.

Time to relax

Not only does relaxation fuel digestion, it literally burns calories. It also creates amazing changes in the body. Since I started meditation a few years ago I have never been slimmer. My emotional issues with food have vanished and I now see it in a different light altogether. I no longer see food as something that is fattening or bad, I see it as a beautiful nourishing gift from nature that gives me daily energy, health and vitality. I also see myself in a different light. Finally, after years of self-criticism, I am able to love myself. It took me 38 years, but I got there in the end.

Often, weight gain is chemical in nature. Some of the most poisonous chemicals you digest do not come from food at all. Rather, they are chemicals you self- produce. It's that dreaded cortisol again, the substance you produce through stress, that is damaging you and piling on the pounds.

Yes, weight gain is about diet and what you eat.

Yet it's also about how you live, how you think and simply how you are. Personally, I'd recommend meditation to anyone. It's wonderful.

It's in the blood

To understand what happens to your food, you also need to know how your blood works. Your blood is set at an alkaline count of 7.365. The pH scale goes from one to 14, with seven being neutral. Anything below seven is acidic and anything above is base or alkaline.

Like your body temperature, your blood is set at a specific level and if it varies from that you experience problems. Your body, therefore, goes to great lengths to maintain its slightly alkaline fluid environment. If it becomes too acidic, your health is compromised and it will tap into its alkalising, buffering reserves to neutralise the acidity and maintain its delicate balance of 7.365.

Some of these alkaline buffers would include calcium from your bones and magnesium from your muscles.

The ratio of acid to alkaline is something else you need to understand. It takes 20 parts of alkalinity to neutralise one part of acidity. This makes investigating an alkalising diet even more key to maintaining your ideal weight and health.

So from here, the most important thing to know and put into practice would be: which foods are acidic; which foods are alkaline? If you could make the most alkalising foods delicious and plentiful in our diets, you would have found the ultimate solution to the weight problems you have today.

I know this to be true from my own experience over the last nine years of studying, living and enjoying this kind of diet. In fact, there is no need to make alkaline foods delicious, as they are already delicious in their own right.

Once you remove all that built-up crap from your tongue, you will start to taste your food properly again.

The chemicals, preservatives, colours, salts and sugars in processed food leave a nasty film on your tongue, desensitising your taste buds. The longer you eat those crap foods, the thicker the film gets. Imagine wrapping your tongue in cling film before you ate your favourite food; it wouldn't taste the same, would it?

This is another reason why so many people overeat. They don't taste their foods, and therefore constantly feel unsatisfied. However, once you start to eat fresh live foods, this nasty film will start to disappear. Take the tongue test now. Whatever the result, I recommend you invest in a tongue scraper and scrape your tongue every time you brush your teeth.

■ TAKE THE TONGUE TEST

Look at your tongue in the mirror. Is it...

- ➤ **Furry? You're toxic!**
- ➤ **Yellow and green? Clean up right now!**
- ➤ **Pink and clean? Great, that's healthy.**

CRAP TO CUT

Foods you should avoid

Right, now let's really get down to it. Don't panic, though, I said foods to avoid; as I told you earlier, no food is actually banned here (well, just one). However, the following all have an acid-forming effect on the body, so if you want to lose weight easily and naturally, you should give them a miss wherever possible. Remember what an acid food does: it converts to an acid ash and your body rushes to the rescue to produce another fat cell to absorb it...that's called weight gain.

Although no food is banned, it's important that you understand the consequences of eating acids and then make your own judgment based on this understanding. These foods have been processed in one way or another. They no longer contain vital energy or enzymes and take more energy from your body to digest than they actually give you. They also have little or no water content. Consequently, eating these foods results in fatigue and compromised health. Before we proceed, think of the word acid; what does it mean to you? Now hold that thought as you read the following:

Coffee. Not so cool

A very strong source of caffeine, coffee is not a food that can be consumed in its raw natural state. It has to go through all sorts of processing before it is palatable and reaches the shelves. Imagine the bitter taste of a coffee bean on your tongue. Drinking too much coffee raises your blood pressure and insulin levels, which in turn make your body store fat. It is a diuretic, so you lose water every time you drink a cup. Coffee beans are roasted and the liquid by-product is used to make instant coffee. Which means what you drink is actually tar.

DDT is an insecticide used on coffee plants that has, thankfully, been banned in the UK and USA, but is still used in countries we import coffee beans from. And why was it banned? Because it's highly poisonous, that's why.

Anything else? Oh, coffee stains your teeth, gives you bad breath and falsely stimulates the adrenal glands. Constantly stimulating the adrenal glands compromises your health and weakens your immune system. It also generates fat cells and is a sure way to a fat, blobby belly.

Imagine the colour of your blood when you have been drinking coffee all day. It looks like a dirty stream. That stream of dirty, acidic liquid is bathing all of the cells in your body and increasing your fat production. So, every single morning you are starting your day with a dose of poison. Nice. If you add artificial sweeteners or dairy products to that poison you will be fat and sick forever.

Would you give a baby a cup of coffee for breakfast? What about your precious pet? Well, why is it OK to give it an adult then? Do you reach a certain age in life when you become immune to poison? Do you heck --it's actually the opposite. The older you get, the more vulnerable you become.

Somewhere along the line, we've stopped valuing our health, and how sad is that? Just look at any coffee drinkers you know. Notice how many of them are overweight. Check out the dark circles under their eyes. Office workers who drink copious amounts all day are classic examples. Study their midriff area in particular.

Almost all of the private clients I see were once huge coffee drinkers. In fact, I know it as soon as they walk into my office. They have an ashen complexion and a weary look around the eyes. Plus, of course, they're carrying too much weight, mostly around their abdomen. I'm delighted to say that when they return a month later, after cutting down or eliminating the coffee, they always looked refreshed, revived and have lost weight. I have never had a client who tells me they have missed coffee. The benefits of health and vitality always taste better than the coffee does.

In truth, we have all been brainwashed into drinking this stuff. It's now trendy and cool. We even walk round holding coffee in paper containers; what's that all about, are we really that desperate? It's very sociable to meet for a coffee or have a cappuccino after a meal. Yet remember when you tried coffee for the first time as a child. Remember how bitter it tasted? Well, it still tastes the same; it's just that you now associate a good feeling with it so somehow it seems to taste better. I have a Labrador dog called Mico. He will eat or drink anything apart from coffee or alcohol. Animals instinctively know a poison; lucky them.

When I was overweight I used to go to Starbucks three to four times a week. I used to order a skinny latte (acid) and a granola bar (sugar, sugar and more sugar). I really thought I was making a healthy choice; no wonder I had a weight problem. After I had eaten the granola bar I would still berate myself for being weak and then spend the rest of the day feeling guilty (producing even more acid). Now I go occasionally and have steamed soya milk with nutmeg and cinnamon, or maybe a peppermint or green tea with honey, all delicious. If it's lunchtime and my body needs food, I have one of their vegetarian wraps. They're nutritious and satisfying, no sugar, no caffeine and no acid. Most importantly, there is no guilt, just enjoyment. I'm relaxed and guilt-free so my body is set for calorie burning, not calorie storing.

My fetish for granola bars ended the day I asked to see the nutritional information available at Starbucks. Guess what? The so called healthy granola bar I had been eating had roughly the same amount of sugar, bad fats and calories as the decadent chocolate cake. I was shocked. How many other people like me were being fooled, I wonder.

There is always an opportunity to make a "better than" choice. I now realise it wasn't the coffee that tempted me to Starbucks; it was the company, the environment and the warm drink. It was also a place where I could escape for an hour. Coffee was just the old association. I now have a new association and make healthier and wiser choices. I still enjoy the experience, in fact I enjoy it more because the whole experience is nourishing for my mind and body. There's more good news, too. The last time I went to Starbucks, I noticed fresh fruit salad and raw almonds in the chiller cabinet. Progress!

That's what this programme is all about, making a better than choice (better than the one you used to make).

Please realise that many of the cups of coffee you drink are really just habit. It's not necessarily the taste or thirst that makes you put the kettle on, it's the association. There is nothing nourishing about eight cups of coffee every day. The other thing to consider, of course, is the more coffee you drink, the less water you drink, and you need water if you want to be slim. Coffee can never quench your thirst because it's a diuretic and actually makes you thirstier.

■ CUT THE CRAP **COFFEE**

> ➤ **Start by reducing the number of cups you have, and replace with hot or tepid water, dandelion coffee, peppermint, green or redbush tea.**
> ➤ **It's not about an addiction; it's more the habit of having a hot drink in your hand.**
> ➤ **Slowly but surely, wean yourself off.**
> ➤ **Increase your water intake between cups.**
> ➤ **Only have a cup when you can really enjoy it. Take time to sit quietly and taste what you are actually drinking.**
> ➤ **Drink a large glass of water with a slice of lime immediately afterwards. Clean your teeth to remove the residue of acid from your tongue.**

You don't have to give coffee up completely. I would never advise you give anything up completely as variety is the spice of life.

I will say that clients who cut out coffee completely not only lose weight faster, but also manage to keep it off more easily. The choice is yours.

Sugar —sweet tooth, saggy tummy

Here is a subject I could write a whole chapter on. In my next book, I most certainly will. The detrimental effects of sugar are too long to list in full here, but we'll start with the two real biggies – premature ageing and obesity. I've been in the health and wellness industry for many years now, and have seen so many times how sugar ages the skin prematurely. A classic symptom of a sugar addict is puffiness around the eyes and jowls. Others are cellulite, loose skin tone, flabby upper arms and water retention. I'm sure my own cellulite is a result of years of sugar addiction.

The obesity scenario is even worse. A hundred years ago, the average person in Britain consumed 5lbs of sugar a year. Now it's 160lbs! Sugar is poison in disguise. It's the biggest contributor to weight gain in the world, bar none. Most people have been hoodwinked to think it's fat that's the problem, when in fact it's sugar. Almost all processed foods have sugar as a main ingredient. Low fat foods, condiments and ready-made meals, including so-called reduced calorie foods, are laden with it. Check food labels; you're in for a shock. Sugar is an acid in disguise. It rots your teeth, your body and your mind. It acts like glue in the body, sticking your cells together. It is instantly stored as fat and is difficult to burn off. Too much sugar causes fatigue, mood swings, depression, lack of concentration, cellulite and cravings. One of the biggest risks of a high sugar diet is diabetes type two, which is now becoming an epidemic.

In a nutshell, I believe that if you don't control your sugar intake you will never control your weight. It's the worst, worst, worst acid you can put in your body. Did I make that clear enough or do you want me to shout it out again?

I said that sugar is found in all processed foods, without exception. This may not surprise you, put like that. But the foods where sugar is used may well do when I spell them out. Foods like soups, processed meat, breads, sauces, diet foods, pastas, tinned vegetables and so many more. Take a look at the ingredients on packets, cartons and tins in your food cupboards and you will be shocked.

And here's the best one of all. They now use sugar on French fries! More later.

Sugar is like crack, and the food manufacturers know it. So does the tobacco industry, with many cigarette brands containing tobacco roasted in the stuff to make it even more addictive. Didn't know that one, did you? There's a lot you don't know. It doesn't say it on the packet, either, but it's there. In my opinion, sugar is more addictive than nicotine.

In its raw state, sugar is indeed a natural food. The pity is we don't get it before it's refined and stripped of all its minerals, enzymes, fibre, vitamins and nutrients. Refined sugar has no nutritional value whatsoever, and yet the food manufacturers shove the stuff into every food at every given opportunity. To make matters worse, it's usually added to food that already contains huge amounts of hideous fat, calories and cholesterol.

Sugar is an inside job. First it wrecks your insides and then it shows up on your outside. Every time you consume sugar, your pancreas immediately has to go to work releasing insulin. If too much sugar is consumed, insulin levels rise and the body stores both the insulin and excess sugar (acid) in the fat cells. The more sugar, the more fat you produce. Believe it: sugar really makes you fat!

Look at the cultures that don't eat sugar, such as the Chinese and Japanese. They tend to be very slim people and do not suffer from cellulite. There is nothing wrong with eating sweet foods; we all love sweet foods. In fact, you have both sweet and salty taste buds on your tongue so you are naturally meant to eat sweet foods.

However, I'm sure Mother Nature didn't give you them so you could get high blood pressure and diabetes. In nature, there is no sweet, poisonous food, only naturally sweet foods that taste good and nourish.

You probably don't need telling that women, in particular, like sweet foods. The word "sweet" is used for many of the things we associate comfort with – sweet love, sweet home, sweet heart. Yet it's not just the taste of sweet foods that appeal; as with coffee, it's the feelings we associate with them.

Kids suffer most

Adults are becoming increasingly aware of the dangers associated with consuming too much sugar. Candida, yeast infections, obesity, depression and mood swings are just a few of the symptoms that have manifested themselves over the past decade. However, it's our children whose health issues are surfacing at an alarming rate, hyperactivity being one of them. Children know no better; they are the innocent victims of sugar addiction.

Even with my wealth of knowledge in nutritional science, I only recently discovered that the "low fat" oven chips my children occasionally have as a treat were soaked in sugar before freezing. Yes, they're now putting sugar on chips! As the label said, they were indeed low fat, for a processed food anyway. Yet nowhere on the package did it say "high in sugar". Silly me, fancy not knowing that! By the way, did you know the fast food chains add sugar to the oil for making fries? No wonder kids love 'em. Finger lickin' good indeed!

What's more, most school dinners are no longer fresh and are loaded with sugar. Vending machines are still ever present in schools, despite the government announcing they would all be removed. Portion sizes have doubled and crisps, chocolate, cakes, biscuits and fizzy drinks are now considered acceptable as an everyday snack. Even worse, parents think they are helping their children by giving them diet drinks. No, no, no! You are making it even worse; not only will they get fat, they'll get sick too.

Call me old fashioned, but wasn't there once a taboo about eating between meals? I clearly remember my parents telling me not to snack because I would ruin my meal. Only 20 years ago these same foods were considered a rare treat. When I was young, the only sugar I was ever allowed was organic honey, purchased from the local bee farm. We had the choice of two types, runny for drinks and solid for toast or sandwiches. Honey is also extremely versatile. It was smeared on our cuts and wounds to accelerate healing. My mother even used it as a facemask, while my father added it to his hot lemon and water. Just going to collect honey was a big event to look forward to, and a wonderful childhood memory. It's still part of my everyday diet.

Here's another memory. Once I found a 20p piece on the pavement. My younger brother Tony and I ran to the local corner shop and immediately bought four Mars Bars. We felt so naughty because sugar was a big no no at home. In those days, my father was probably considered a health freak because he cared about our health. We grew fruit and vegetables in the garden, and our breakfast was often grapes from the greenhouse. Anyway, the Mars Bars were such a treat and I can still remember our excitement. I ate one of mine on the way home and the other was saved for the following weekend. I hid it under my bed and looked at it every day. Nowadays, confectionary isn't a treat for the majority of children, just something they eat every day without considering the consequences.

Unfortunately, due to a chain of disastrous events, by the age of 12 we were orphaned and let out into the big wide world of sugar. Because I had been deprived of it, I went mad and ate it at every given opportunity. By the age of 14 I was most definitely a sugar addict, and my weight issue was starting to become evident. All that sugar had pitched a tent on my hips, thighs and cheeks. The negative feelings associated with sugar made me eat secretly, and to this day I still feel guilty when I eat something sweet. Even today, when I go through anything traumatic I still revert to secret eating. It's my "self-sabotage" pattern.

Keep your children sweet

Today, I have a more relaxed approach to sugar with my own children. I don't buy anything processed, so our fridge and cupboards only contain fresh foods. We have lots of fruit, nuts, seeds, honey, soya yoghurts, smoothies and occasionally I treat them to a bar of halva. So if they need anything sweet at home there's lots of good fresh stuff to choose from. If they choose biscuits, cakes and chocolate when they're out, that's up to them. At weekends I make flapjacks and they go down a storm. Every morning, I send them off to school with a bottle of water and a snack such as a sesame or fruit and nut bar, and occasionally a fresh smoothie. If they don't want it, they leave it, but there's no crap on offer.

I know from my own experience that deprivation only creates desire, so I try not to set too many rules that are only going to be broken. My kids are normal kids. I would be naive to think they don't ever indulge in processed crap. Of course they do, but not at home, which is the biggest part of their lives. I hope my example will have an influence. It's the best I can do, and the same goes for you. My parents' influence certainly worked on me. My biggest challenge is other people feeding my kids crap; it's a difficult one.

If I ever get the chance to meet Jamie Oliver, I know I will just have to run up to him and kiss him! I'm eternally thankful for his hard work in changing awareness of how our children are eating. If ever anyone deserved a knighthood, it's Jamie. He has fought tirelessly to get the government to accept that change has to start with school meals. Our children are the future. If things don't change drastically, then the long-term effects are going to be devastating.

Obesity in children is now rising every day and overwhelmingly it's sugar that's causing the problem. Recently, I read some reports that disturbed me for weeks. Over half of all Americans are overweight and out of shape, but children are going downhill fastest of all. In fact, according to the Center for Disease Control and Prevention, if things don't change, one out of every three children born this year will eventually develop type-two diabetes. This is a chronic illness that leads to a host of crippling conditions, including blindness, asthma, heart disease, depression and even death. I might not live in the USA, but children are children wherever they live and they deserve better than this. What's more, historically, whatever happens in the US inevitably filters through to Britain. Perhaps most sobering of all, this is the first generation likely to be outlived by their parents.

Manufacturers are deliberately putting additives into food that are proven to be addictive, and eventually our children will die because of it. If everyday I put a little arsenic in your tea and you ultimately became ill and died, wouldn't I be responsible? Are they not both cases of premeditated manslaughter? In my mind, they are. We all have to sit up, open our eyes, ears and mouths and start taking responsibility for what we put in our own bodies, and even more importantly, our children's. Stop relying on the advice of strangers and make it your business to read the food labels before you poison your own kids.

A word for diabetics

Having both friends and family with the condition, I've had firsthand experience of watching diabetics eat. I call it a "condition" because I know diabetes type two can be completely reversed by diet alone. I have seen it with my own eyes on no less than four occasions.

By the way, have you noticed how some diabetics seem to tie up their whole identity with their condition? You meet them and they say, "I am a diabetic." Have you ever heard anyone say "Hi, I'm a hay fever sufferer"? It's nonsense! If people tell me, "I am a diabetic", I always tell them "No, you are not a diabetic, you just suffer from diabetes". Diabetes is a condition, not who you are.

The symptoms of diabetes type two present themselves as an illness, and many can be debilitating. The constant fatigue means the person is always focused on the condition, and as you know, "where intention goes, energy flows". As I've said, though, almost all of these symptoms can be totally reversed and cured.

What's clear is that diabetics will go to great lengths to avoid obvious sugars such as sweets, pastries and confectionary, but many will continue to eat hidden sugars like white bread, pasta, tomato ketchup, wine, potatoes, cheese and bacon. Often they'll even drink diet coke. They will also go so far as to decline a piece of chewing gum because of its sugar content, yet continue to drink alcohol.

I know this is due to lack of information and education, and therefore I'm asking that if you know a diabetic, perhaps you'd care to share this information with them. After all, it could change or even save their lives. If you want to know more about how diet can reverse diabetes, read *There Is A Cure For Diabetes* by Gabriel Cousins.

■ CUT THE CRAP **SUGAR**

> ➤ **Try to avoid all processed sugar and instead substitute with Manuka honey or better still agave nectar, a sweet natural syrup. They are both delicious and nourishing at the same time.**

> ➤ **Manuka's immunity enhancing benefits have now resulted in it being given to cancer patients in hospitals to prevent them contracting the super bug MRSA. It's almost the only food in the world that never goes off.**

> ➤ **And if you really like sweet, processed foods, don't try to eliminate them completely; denial only leads to desire. Enjoy a little of what you fancy now and again and eat without guilt. It's the dosage that's the poison.**

> ➤ **Don't fall for sugars in disguise: fructose, sucrose, dextrose. Anything ending with "ose" is usually a sugar.**

Artificial sweetener: man-made suicide

ARTIFICIAL SWEETENERS ARE POISON. THEY MAKE YOU fat. And they're suicidal for diabetics. Now, do I continue with the commercial? In truth, nothing artificial should ever be put in a natural body. Yet aspartame, the number one artificial sweetener, is found in almost every sugar-free product, diet food and other branded sweetener. It's also commonly known as the "silent killer".

Now, that's got you interested, hasn't it? Well, would you be surprised to learn that the additive you probably feed your kids and yourself was actually made as a chemical for biological warfare? Now it's going to war on your body, slowly and surely destroying each cell.

The US military spent $millions researching and developing aspartame, so when they didn't use it themselves, they had to find something else to do with it. That something was to put it in our foods and drinks. Believe me, this stuff is absolute, utter crap. No, it's worse. It's literally poison.

Right now, you're probably thinking "You're kidding me!" Well, I wish I was, but I'm not. This is one of the most lethal substances on the planet and we are giving it to our children. As if getting sick isn't bad enough, most people consume it because they are trying to lose weight or have been brainwashed to believe it's better than sugar. Wrong again! This crap that makes you fat, tired and sick has been linked to Alzheimer's, cancer, memory loss, muscle wastage, hyperactivity and birth defects, to name just a few. The symptoms of aspartame poisoning can also mimic those of multiple sclerosis, so millions of people all over the world are being wrongly diagnosed and sentenced to a lifetime of fear and unnecessary pharmaceutical drugs. Right now, make the decision never to put this stuff in your body again. If you do, you might as well drip feed yourself with arsenic.

(I know I said I never say "never", but I make no apologies for making an exception in this case.)

100 times sweeter than the real thing, artificial sweeteners work by tricking the pancreas into thinking sugar is on its way. This in turn raises insulin levels and therefore increases your risk. It's also why diabetics should never eat foods containing this poison. Elevated insulin levels lead to the production of fat, particularly around the midriff.

As I've indicated, people who eat diet foods unknowingly consume vast amounts of aspartame. Ironically, it actually causes the body to store fat, and has the reverse of the desired effect. There has been no recorded evidence that sweeteners help weight loss, not one scientific paper. So every time you think you are being "good" and drinking a diet soda, eating a sugar free yoghurt or even drinking one of those crappy flavoured waters, you are actually perpetuating your weight problem, not solving it.

So many people who consume this crap constantly complain about sweet cravings – then go and binge on sugar or carbs! It's the sweeteners that are causing the cravings. How clever the food industry is. Listen: sweeteners make you fat. Have you got that now?

Lets face it, if this crap actually worked we would all be slim. But that's not the case, is it? The truth is that millions of people have been drinking and eating copious amounts of the stuff for years and getting fatter.

People seem to think if they order a chocolate brownie and then swill it down with a diet soda it somehow makes it better. I have asked hundreds of clients why they continue to drink this stuff; the answer is always the same. "Well, if I drink a diet soda with my meal, even if the meal is fattening, I reckon I'm saving some calories." Saving calories for what, to eat more? It's a ridiculous notion because, as I have said, this stuff simply makes you crave sweet foods and then overeat later on in the day. Do the maths, your calories count goes up, not down.

If you must continue to drink liquid shit, my advice to you is to drink the real McCoy. Even the demon sugar is better than those man-made chemicals they dare to call sweeteners. When these diet drinks and sodas first came on the market they were faced with enormous resistance, especially from people not needing to lose weight. They tasted bitter, sharp and left a strange tang on the tongue. Well, they still taste the same. All that's happened is that millions of pounds of advertising have brainwashed you into believing that the benefits outweigh the taste and bingo, soon you acquired a taste for it! Diet Coke adverts, for example, are now sexy and sporty. This is the fastest way to seduce women and children, their target markets. If your want weak bones, drink this stuff. It leaches calcium from our bones, the evidence is the rising numbers of adolescent osteoporosis.

If we can be brainwashed to like the taste of cigarettes, coffee and alcohol, we can be brainwashed to like anything. Take the example of someone who used to drink two or three lumps of sugar in their tea and then gives it up for health reasons. If by mistake a few grains of sugar are now put into their tea, they grimace and even spit it out, appalled by the taste. That's how powerfully our minds work if we decide we no longer like something. Beware, aspartame is now a $1 billion dollar industry and is being cleverly disguised as Splenda, Equal, Canderal, Sweetex and many more brands.

Before being finally accepted in America by the FDA (Food and Drug Administration),- aspartame was denied eight times owing to the fact it had disastrous effects on the human body and brain. Some of the 92 side effects of aspartame listed by the FDA include memory loss, Alzheimer's, blindness, brain lesions, joint pain, food cravings, weight gain, depression and birth defects.

Eventually, after a period of around 23 years, during which medical reports had been manipulated and some very big guns indeed wheeled out to lobby for the cause, aspartame was approved for use without restriction in 1996. Gobsmacked? I know I was – and still am. How does a poison become not a poison? It doesn't seem to matter to the manufacturers. It's all about money, money, money -- not your health, nor your children's.

I'm also incredibly frustrated that doctors will happily give a patient insulin but not the simple advice, "Don't use sweeteners". This is a food even I wouldn't dare tell you to enjoy with moderation. After all, who am I to gamble with your life?

We are a genetic experiment in the process. We will not know the long-term effects of these products until the damage is done. In my opinion, anything that tastes so bitter must be a poison. Just put a sweetener on your tongue and see how it tastes and feels. The bitterness is the acid. So many people have been poisoned by aspartame that there are now victim support groups across the globe. There have been more complaints about this product that any other in the world.

Organic what?

I just heard that Coca Cola are about to launch an organic version of the drink. They call it organic and we are led to believe it's good for us? The sad thing is that parents will give their kids this stuff with a clear conscience...oh dear.

Let me remind you, organic must be raw organic to be of any health benefit; it has to have grown. Have you seen any coca cola fields lately? The stuff in the can that's labeled "organic", forget it. Save your money and buy the regular brand. Organic in a can? You've got to be joking!

■ DAIRY DON'T DO IT

YOU THINK YOU GET YOUR CALCIUM FROM DAIRY products? Think again! I don't blame you for believing this myth; after all, we were brought up on the stuff and surely we wouldn't be given something at school that was unhealthy, would we? Prepare yourself now because this section is going to challenge your years of brainwashing more than any other.

Dairy products, especially milk, are to be avoided. They are highly acidic and lifeless, as well as being mucus-forming. The lactose in milk is sugary. If you think of how big and how quickly a calf grows when fed only on cow's milk, it's no wonder that dairy products have been linked to obesity. The average calf is born weighing only 90lbs, yet ends up over 1,000lbs within six short months. That's how fattening dairy is!

It has nothing to do with the calorie content, it's our inability to digest dairy that's the problem. After the age of three, most human beings stop producing up to 90% of the essential enzymes required to digest milk, rennin and lactase. Research has revealed that 20% of Caucasian children and 80% of black children have neither of the required enzymes in their intestines; no wonder milk is up there with the top three allergies. The caisin in cow's milk is 100 times greater than mother's milk and unsuitable for human digestion. Put simply, you're not designed to digest your own mother's breast milk after the age of around three, never mind that of a cow.

What's more, the undigested lactose, added growth hormones and acidic nature of pasteurised milk encourage the growth of bacteria in your intestines. An over-acidic environment contributes to a greater risk of cancer, because tumours need acid to thrive and grow. There has always been a direct correlation between breast cancer and the consumption of dairy products. Again, you only have to look at countries such as Japan and China, where dairy is not consumed and the rate of breast cancer is very low.

Bring on the sub

By changing to soya or oat milk fortified with vitamin D, calcium and isoflavoids, you immediately reduce your risk of all cancers, in particular breast and prostate, by a whopping 33%. So what are you waiting for? I lost more than two stones over a period of two years. The last stone came off the fastest, when I finally stopped being stubborn and dropped dairy in all forms, including cheese, yoghurt and cream.

Like everybody else, I had been hoodwinked from childhood into believing that drinking milk was one of the healthiest things on earth. My father used to make me drink full cream Jersey milk, morning and night. The stuff was like drinking single cream and loaded with saturated fat. However, fattening it may have been, but it wasn't full of growth hormones and steroids and the cows were organic clover fed. Milk was different back then.

Since childhood, I had always suffered from the nasal condition rhinitis while my brother suffered badly from tonsillitis and sinusitis. Our problems were compounded by the fact that milk is probably the worst culprit for causing over production of mucus in children. Sad to say, in my ignorance I did the same thing as my father with my own children. My eldest son developed eczema, and my youngest always had a runny nose.

Fortunately, all this has now changed. When I dropped the dairy, not only did I drop 14lbs of fat, but also my nasal condition. It disappeared for good. More great news is that soya is available almost everywhere now, and is even being advertised on national TV. Soya milk has improved over the years; it's now delicious and tastes a little bit like vanilla milkshake. Soya yoghurts are thick, creamy, yummy and satisfying and children love them. My favourite is So Good. Soya cheese is a great substitute and a permanent fixture in my fridge.

Apparently, the large dairy manufacturers are now buying up the soya product companies, which suggests they must be panicking and making a Plan B. As more and more people wise up to the lies about diary and the truth about soya, we're going to witness a huge influx of soya products in our major supermarkets and grocery stores. Of course, we will never be told that dairy is bad for us, just that soya is better. Be prepared, though. Before the government accept soya as being healthy, the dairy industry will do their level best to manipulate the truth and condemn it.

Another alternative is almond milk that is also delicious. It's more expensive than soya and currently not widely available in the supermarkets. Rice milk tastes good too, but is much thinner in consistency. Oatly is in the middle and a big favourite with my clients; it's high in calcium and very low in fat and sugar.

Whose breast is best?

Every species on this planet was gifted with unique, perfectly matching milk that is available the moment babies are born. Baby seals drink seal milk. Kittens drink cat milk. Puppies drink dog milk. Baby elephants drink elephant milk, and I'm sure you see where this is going. Once the infant is weaned, they never, ever go back to drinking from the breast again. So why are you drinking from a cow's breast, when you were weaned from your own mother's breast so long ago?

Oh, and while we're at it, why is it OK to drink from a cow but not a cat, a pig or even your pet dog? You could just as easily put sheep's milk in your cuppa or skunk's milk on your muesli. Chimpanzees are our nearest relative and 99% of their DNA is the same as ours, so shouldn't we be drinking their milk, if anybody's?

If you had to go and suck the stuff out of the cow yourself, would you still go for it? I doubt it very much. The thought of drinking another human being's breast milk makes people sick, so why is it fine to drink a dirty big beast's milk? Human breast milk is sterile, and can be drunk directly from the breast without any further sterilisation. It is the perfect nutrient for the human body, and has all the essential nutrients a baby needs in its first few months of life. This is the most important period as it's the time we have our biggest growth spurt and our skeletal system grows and strengthens. But, if it were sold in the supermarket and branded as "Supermilk", would you consider drinking it? No chance!

Cows have been carefully selected because the poor beasts are the ones who produce the most milk. Their tanks (udders) are the biggest, so it makes them commercially viable. This is the one and only reason we drink cow's milk. It's a commercial decision. It's not because their mammary juice gives us the most nutritional benefits, just that they are docile, gentle creatures that happen to produce and store the most milk. They conform easily and don't fight back. They don't bite or attack, they just obey. The unnatural process the poor things go through to give us a sticky white substance that creates mucus, clogs up our bodies and makes us fat and sick is cruel and extremely painful. A cow would never hurt us, so why are we hurting them?

We have been psychologically manipulated by the dairy industry, and ruled by fear to keep drinking milk. There is no more effective advertising strategy than to convince people they will become ill without using a product. This is how the dairy industry works. They frighten people into thinking their bones will become brittle, and prey on women, particularly the pre-menopausal. The threat of osteoporosis looms over us like a guillotine. You only have to go to a baby clinic and see all the adverts for milk – all financed by the dairy industry. A mother is made to believe giving her child milk is the only way to health. I was one of those mothers who bought into that crap.

You may be familiar with the slogans "Milk's Gotta Lotta Bottle" and "DrinkaPintaMilkaDay". How about "Milk makes strong teeth and bones"? Wrong, wrong, wrong!

We are one of the largest consumers of dairy in the world, and yet we have one of the highest rates of brittle bones and osteoporosis. Something's clearly not adding up here, folks!

Duh! The four countries that consume the largest amounts of dairy in the world are the USA, Great Britain, Sweden and Finland. The four countries with the highest incidence of osteoporosis are, you guessed it, the USA, Great Britain, Sweden and Finland. Africa and Asia consume the least, and they also happen to have the lowest incidence of osteoporosis. Now, it's not rocket science to see where this is going.

When I was young, I took a career break to travel around the world. I worked with British Airways as a stewardess for a while.

I frequently did the routes to Japan and China, and spent a lot of time talking to passengers – and believe me, I can talk for England! I was left in no doubt that Chinese and Japanese people don't like dairy. In fact, they find it repulsive. They describe it as foul smelling and sickly tasting, and simply can't understand why we drink it. They also say that British people smell of sour milk. Nice.

Osteoporosis is so rare in China that they don't even have a word for it in their language. They have the world's biggest population and the lowest rates of this debilitating condition. Personally, I can't stand the smell of milk now, it makes me sick too. No amount of celebrity-endorsed advertising is going to deny the truth. The truth is that clearly you don't need dairy to get calcium for your bones. Please tell me you are convinced now. If not, go and stand in your common sense corner and have a good talk with yourself until you are.

Mother Nature's got calcium

If Mother Nature provided us with everything around us so we could survive without cooking, hunting, shopping or preserving, do you really think she would have forgotten to give us essential nutrients like calcium? If milk was our only source of calcium, we would all still be sucking on our mother's breast right now. Can you imagine how inconvenient that would be, having to leave a board meeting to have a suckle? Having to take our mothers on holiday with us would be a nightmare. We would be enslaved to a lifetime of being with our mums.

And what if they died, would we have to suck someone else's mother's breast?

Of course not! We have a ready supply of calcium, like every other nutrient, vitamin and mineral we need for the rest of our lives. Nature is superior to anything else we could ever imagine and never neglects our needs. We don't need to capture or hurt any other species, we just need to look at the food of the land. Everything that grows from the ground has calcium in it.

Actually, the notion that we get all our calcium and vitamin D requirements from milk is another huge lie we've been brainwashed to believe. It makes me angry because so many innocent people have bought this and are now suffering the consequences. If you just trust the information you're given and rely solely on dairy for your calcium, you then become complacent and don't look anywhere else to get this crucial mineral. And that can lead to calcium deficiency, brittle bones and osteoporosis.

■ LOVELY LINDA'S STORY

ON THE TRAIN TO MANCHESTER ONE DAY, I GOT TALKING to a lovely lady called Linda. Linda was three stone overweight and told me she had spent most of her life on a low fat diet. When we spoke I could see the frustration in her face as she told me she did all the right things, everything the doctor had advised and still couldn't lose weight. When I asked her what she ate every day she promptly told me. (This is a trait of people overweight; they always know what they eat and what they plan to eat because they are so obsessed with food. Ask a slim person and they will rarely remember because it isn't important to them…ah ha, do they have a secret?)

Proudly, Linda told me she had at least one and a half pints of semi skimmed milk a day, two low fat yogurts and cheese with her sandwich at lunch time. I had a light bulb moment and immediately suggested she reduce the amount of dairy in her diet and consider switching to soya or rice milk, I felt sure that was her problem. I had barely got the word "problem" out of my mouth when I got that familiar face of resistance It's a bit like a porcupine raising its spikes (you get used to that in my job). "Oh no," she said – rather, she shouted, "I couldn't do that, I suffer from osteoporosis and my doctor says I need lots and lots of dairy!" There was a pause, then I replied, "How long have you suffered from that condition, Linda? "Three years," she replied. "And how long have you been drinking dairy?" "All my life, "she answered. "My father was a milk man." There wasn't enough time left on that train journey for me to go into the whys and hows, so I offered Linda a free session so I could offer my help. It turned out that Linda's condition was hereditary – or so she thought; her mother had suffered from the same thing. As far as I'm concerned, the only thing hereditary was her eating habits.

Five months later, Linda has lost 32lbs and is feeling healthier than ever and her GP called me to ask me to send him a copy of my programme. Funnily enough, he told me he was overweight and suffered from high cholesterol, both conditions caused by consuming the wrong foods. I couldn't resist the opportunity to offer him a free consultation; he hasn't accepted yet but I'm hopeful. It's all about education, folks; it's about thinking out of the box and using common sense. If drinking mammary juice feels right for you then go for it, it's your choice at the end of the day.

If you really must get your calcium from a cow, it would make more sense to eat its bones and teeth than suck off its mammary glands. Do cows drink milk to get their own calcium? No, they eat grass, and lots of it. Green plant foods are one of the richest sources of calcium you'll find. What about the African elephant, the largest animal in the bush? It takes tons of calcium to form those huge tusks, teeth and toenails, so do they need to drink milk? No, of course not, they eat vegetation. What about the chicken that lays an egg every day? The shell is made of calcium, so do chickens drink milk? Getting the picture now?

Contrary to popular belief, cows don't ever need to be milked – their udders, just like women's breasts, exist even when there's no milk in them – while the process of manufacturing milk and unnaturally milking them with electric pumps creates many nasty infections such as mastitis. To treat these infections and prevent illnesses that might slow down production, cows are routinely given large doses of medication and antibiotics. These pass though into the milk and into your glass. In fact, this is one of the main reasons so many people are becoming immune to antibiotics.

Once the milk industry has finished with the cows for dairy purposes, they are slaughtered for their meat value. To ensure the size of the animal is commercially viable, they are given growth hormones that again pass down, to us. This is the main reason children are reaching puberty early.

Honestly, milk sucks. Big time.

Despite what you have been hoodwinked into believing, it has nothing going for it whatsoever. Milk allergies are now listed among the top three allergies in the world. They have been linked to conditions as varied as eczema, asthma, sinusitis and arthritis. Treating these in isolation is like pulling up weeds without using weed killer: a pointless exercise, because the symptoms, like the weeds, will always return. You need to address the cause and stop drinking milk.

For the reasons I've given above, milk is no longer given out in schools to infant children. Cow's milk was definitely made for infants – calves! No other species in the world drinks another species' milk, and humans were never intended to drink cow's milk. The other thing you might like to consider is the way commercial cows are raised. Cows are naturally vegetarians. They graze on grass all day to acquire their nutritional requirements. Yet commercial practice involves feeding cattle on animal fodder. Like humans, they were never designed to eat meat. If you still want to drink cow's milk after all this, at least buy the organic brands, from cows that have been able to wander freely and eat clover grass as Mother Nature intended. Boiling it first will make easier to digest.

Drop the dairy – lose the pounds

Dairy products are extremely high in fat and cholesterol and devoid of fibre – the opposite of what any health expert would recommend. It is widely accepted that best for the human body is a naturally low fat and high fibre diet.

So do yourself a massive favour. Drop dairy and I guarantee you will drop unwanted pounds too. As you've seen, an acidic diet that contains animal products, meat, cooked food and dairy, creates an acidic pH in the blood. To neutralise these acids and rebalance the blood, your body calls upon stored calcium from bones and magnesium from muscles. The more acidic your diet, the weaker your bones and muscles become. This may explain why many middle-aged women are prone to flabby muscles and brittle bones.

Calcium intake is only half of the story; calcium loss is the other. This is one of the main reasons we shrink as we get older. Do you really think it was Mother Nature's plan to send us back into the ground as we get older by shrinking us? Not at all. In cultures where bone density is strong, loss of height is minimal. Here in the UK it's a different story.

···➤ *If you want to look like a cow, keep drinking like a calf.*
Although remember, even a calf can't survive on cooked milk!

■ CUT THE CRAP **MEAT**

Animal flesh is not the protein source we have been brought up to believe it is. You are whatever you eat eats!

Now, madam, would you like some growth hormone, steroids and antibiotics to go with that chicken breast? Or how about all of these, plus some extra bovine with your steak?

No? Well, I'm afraid to tell you that unless you are buying organic, free range meat and you know its source, that's exactly what you're getting.

"Meat", which refers to any animal that once had a mother or a face, has virtually no nutritional value whatsoever. It contains practically no essential nutrients, and is only 25% protein. The one thing it does have in its favour is vitamin B12, which can also be found in the soil that covers vegetables and fermented foods.

There is a common misconception that red meat is a good protein source. This is simply not true. There are tons more protein in seeds and nuts. Red meat is high in saturated fat and can take as long as 72 hours to digest. During this period, your body's energy levels are depleted and your metabolic rate slowed down. The steroids and growth hormones that are injected into animal flesh are highly acidic and mucus forming, while the antibiotics filter through to your body too. Meat eaters are more likely to suffer with fatigue, flatulence, obesity and poor digestion. Meat is a "dead food" and therefore depletes your body of energy. Red meat also puts a strain on your ability to produce enzymes and hydrochloric acid, which is necessary for digestion.

Contrary to general belief, you have few enzymes to break down meat. Good job too because, if you did, you'd break down your own stomach and intestines. If you chopped up a human being and gave yourself a nice steak, you wouldn't know the difference. It looks the same because it is. Red, dead flesh. Work this out for yourself, you would be self-digesting if you could digest meat.

The growth hormones now injected into meat to plump it up and increase its commercial value also have the same effect on the human body. This is thought to be one reason why young girls are reaching puberty earlier and women are facing premature menopause.

Meat is also very low frequency food, which explains the fatigue and lethargy. What does a lion do after it eats? It sleeps for hours and hours. How do you feel after a Sunday roast? Raring to go or ready to sleep? Our digestive tracts are very long, on average 27 feet, so meat takes over two days to work its way down. Lions, on the other hand, have a digestive tract of only 4 feet.

As I've mentioned, the body has to produce hydrochloric acid to try and break down meat. Animals have five times more than humans, making meat a perfect choice for them – and a lousy one for you. Unless, of course you don't mind walking around with rotting flesh inside your body for two to three days. It gets worse, too. Meat turns to an acid in your intestines, and you start to marinate from the inside out. You use acid to tenderise your meat, don't you? Processed meats such as salami, pepperoni, bacon, chicken, turkey and ham are also loaded with salt, sugar colourings and much more crap. Go out of your way to avoid them.

During my years as a colonic therapist, I have treated patients recovering from bowel cancer who were all strongly advised to avoid meat. Eating meat more than three times a week, and this includes chicken, increases your risk of colon cancer by 50%, the third biggest killer in the UK. It also increases your risk of many other cancers, too. If you must eat meat, make sure you chew it thoroughly and eat a big raw salad to aid digestion.

It's significant that the largest, strongest animals in the jungle, such as the silverback gorilla and the African elephant, are vegetarians. Their body mass requires them to consume high volumes of protein every day, and where do you think they obtain this protein? Yes, good old reliable plant foods, nuts and seeds. There is no such thing as protein deficiency in the wild, and I have never heard of a case in humans either. On average, most people consume four times too much protein, which is a precursor to cancer. If I had a pound for every time someone asked me where I get my protein I'd be a very rich lady. Why, oh why have we been brainwashed to think that the only form of protein available is a dead animal? Just shows how limited our thinking is.

A meal fit for a king?

Another interesting fact is that carnivores on the whole do not eat other carnivores, but prefer to hunt and eat herbivores. Elephants and lions are the "kings" of the jungle, because nothing apart from man threatens their extinction. So they have a free choice to eat whatever creature they fancy. And what do they choose? Elephants eat vegetation and lions eat herbivores. Do they know something we don't?

When a lion kills his prey, the first thing he does is rip out the intestines. His three-course meal consists of:

> **Starter.** The stomach, which contains nuts, seeds and vegetation.
> **Main course.** The small intestine, then the large intestine, both still containing the last plant-based meal the animal ate.
> **Dessert.** The organs such as the liver, lungs and heart, as they contain the highest water content and he's a thirsty boy. All that hunting is hard going!

Normally, by the time he reaches dessert, the rest of the pride are tucking into the carcass, which is considered the least nutritional part of the animal. So even a lion knows where to get the most important nutrients for his diet. In reality, carnivores are not exclusively meat eaters they have a balanced diet.

Vultures are exclusive meat eaters, who eat anything that's already dead. Their diet consists of rotting flesh, no vegetation and little water content. And that saying "You are what you eat" suits them perfectly, doesn't it?

What's in a name?

I wonder. If meat were called "cow", "pig", "hen" or "sheep" would you still eat it? I doubt it very much. If all you had to do was go out and kill one animal with your bare hands to secure an abundance of animal flesh for the rest of your life, could you do that? Would you do it? Thought not.

It's simply not in our nature to eat animals. We are a nation of animal lovers and go out of our way to protect them. After all, we have them as pets, don't we? As Harvey Diamond says, "Give a child a rabbit and an apple. If he plays with the apple and eats the rabbit, I'll eat my hat."

Anyway, even if you could pluck up the courage to kill an animal, how would you catch it? Imagine for a minute that you were back in the Stone Age. First, you would have to find your quarry, which could mean a long walk. Then you'd have to catch it, which would be difficult as you'd have no tools – most animals are fast and squirmy. Let's hope in the process you don't get killed yourself. Next, you would have to tear the flesh open, even more of a challenge as you have no claws. You would have to bite through the fur, then you'd tear into the flesh with your teeth. A few fangs would come in handy, but Mother Nature didn't provide us with those, did she? Fur balls in your throat could also be a problem.

And finally, when you've accomplished all this, how would you digest your prize, without hydrochloric acid? No, that's right: you can't. And because you can't preserve or store it, the flies and maggots would set in pretty fast as well. Which means you would have to repeat the whole process in the next few days. And the few days after that.

Can you imagine putting yourself through all this every time your stomach started to rumble? Of course you can't. Only an idiot would even consider all this palaver when all you have to do is bend, stretch and gather all the plentiful natural food around you. Today, most of us can't even be bothered cooking, never mind hunting! In the spring, when you're walking down a country lane and see a newborn lamb, does your mouth start to water? Or do you feel overwhelmed by its cuteness? Let's face it, we were never designed to eat meat any more than we were meant to eat filings to get iron! Undo the brain washing and decide for yourself.

■ SLAUGHTER OF THE INNOCENTS

I call myself a "flexitarian". By this I mean I never eat red meat, very seldom eat chicken and occasionally eat fish. The majority of the time I eat a plant-based diet, sometimes vegan, sometimes vegetarian. As you know, I am not big on rules or willpower when it comes to food, so I never deprive myself of anything. I did all that nonsense in my dieting days and it never worked.

I listen to my body and have a little of what I fancy and what it needs. I suggest you do the same. I made the decision to stop eating red meat fifteen years ago when I opened my ears and eyes and witnessed the cruelty animals were suffering just so I could eat. It seemed needless when there were so many other, healthier options available. At that time, I was brainwashed to believe that chickens roamed around blissfully on farmyards so I continued to eat them. Maybe that's what I wanted to believe at the time. Now I know better. The health benefits and my desire to keep fit and slim are, of course, major factors in my decision not to eat animal flesh. Yet the primary one is the cruelty to animals, both before and during the slaughter process.

For this reason, writing this next section has been very upsetting for me. My aim is not to upset you, however, just to make you more aware of what is really going on in those slaughterhouses. As the late – and wonderful – Linda McCartney said "If slaughterhouses were made of glass, no one would eat meat". I will spare you most of the details and just give an overview here. If you want to know more, there are many websites including peta.org so please take the time to check them out.

More animals are abused and killed painfully on factory farms and in slaughterhouses than anywhere else on the planet. Tiny chicks have their sensitive beaks cut off with a burning hot blade, and millions of chickens are scalded to death fully conscious in de-feathering tanks every year. Mother pigs are forcibly impregnated in filthy metal crates so small and hard that they can't even turn around or lie down comfortably. Piglets' teeth, tails and testicles cut off without any painkillers.

Workers kneel on ducks to hold them down, shove a hard tube down their throats to force-feed them and enlarge their liver. This is an excruciatingly painful existence, all to make the delicacy foie gras. How this can be a delicacy I will never understand. Ducks cannot scream or shed a tear, but the fear in their faces says it all. By the same token, calves are taken away from their mother, kept in the dark and put in pens where they're unable to lie down or even turn around. They're also forced to stand in their own excrement. All this so we can have a white coloured beef called veal. What is wrong with people who knowingly eat this stuff?

Cattle endure castration, branding and dehorning, all without any pain relief. Many end up being skinned alive or having their hooves cut off while they are still fully conscious. The screams of panic-stricken animals can be heard from far and wide, and abattoir workers wear protective gear to block out the noise. Ever wondered why these places are in the middle of nowhere? These animals can feel pain, panic and despair just as we can, yet are treated without an ounce of compassion. The poor creatures are filled with fear from the moment they step into the slaughterhouse until their suffering finally ends with death. Remember, too, that the fear causes adrenaline and cortisone to flood the meat that you eat, both highly poisonous chemicals known to cause heart disease.

As if the fear and death weren't enough, possibly the worst aspect of all is the sadistic way many workers treat the animals. These people are very poorly paid and morale is low, so they have a grudge against both employer and animal. And if you thought these places were clean, think again. Workers have admitted urinating over animals and regularly vomit on the floors and gulleys. (You and I would vomit if we were there, too.) In her book, *Slaughterhouse*, Gail Eisnitz, Chief Investigator for the Humane Farming Association, interviewed dozens of slaughterhouse workers. Every single one admitted to abusing, torturing and neglecting the animals. Here are just a couple of the more mild quotes, even so, not for the squeamish:

> *"I seen them take those stunners, they are about a yard long, and shove it up the hog's ass...they do it with the cows too... and in their eyes, ears, down their throat, they will be squealing and they just shove it right down there."*

> *"Pigs have come up to me and nuzzled me like a puppy. Two minutes later I had to kill them, beat them to death with a pipe."*

There have been many other reports by undercover investigators revealing even worse accounts than the ones you've just read. Many include sexual abuse, and are just too distressing for me to reveal. I've said what I've said because I couldn't write this book without giving you the true picture. This was my promise from the off.

If you still wish to eat meat, kosher is the "better than" choice. At least the animals are kept in a cruelty free environment and the moment of death is much quicker and less painful for the poor animal. Also, the blood is drained from it so it is cleaner, while the animal has to be free of disease before it is slaughtered.

■ PROCESSED FOODS PROCESSED TO MAKE YOU FAT

I know you have heard this advice before, but do you really understand the implications of eating processed foods? Probably not, which is why you innocently keep consuming them. So let me give you the facts, the real truth, and then you might start to think differently. A processed food is "any food that is not in its natural state". Whether it be frozen, tinned, dried, bottled, sweetened or impregnated with salt and additives, this processing usually has three main harmful side effects:

1. **It kills the nutrients**
2. **It reduces the vitally important water content**
3. **It adds toxins. Yummy!**

We'll take the first one first.

Nutrients. Because these foods have been interfered with, they no longer contain vital nutrients, vitamins and minerals, and therefore do not satisfy hunger. This is why, despite being full, you can still continue to eat them. Remember the famous advert for that savoury snack, "Once you start you just can't stop"? Well, the punch line hits the nail on the head. Many of these foods contain additives that are designed to make you want more. Eating processed foods leads to overeating. Period. If you don't feel full and your body hasn't had the nutrients required to rebuild cells and tissues, it will send a false hunger signal to prompt you to keep eating even when you're not hungry. This is why people who eat mainly processed foods are fat and constantly grazing. Cows graze, and look at the size of that beast. Graze all day and you'll end up looking like a bloated beast yourself.

Throughout all my years of seeing hundreds of private clients, I have never yet had anyone admit to bingeing on a whole bowl of apples, five melons or ten bananas. It just doesn't happen. Why? Because a natural food such as a melon, apple or banana is nutritionally dense and gives you all the nutrients you need. It's Mother Nature's own package food. It's also a natural convenience food, all you have to do is wash it and off you go. There is no need to keep chomping and chomping; after just one portion you feel satisfied.

The Ds have it! Fresh foods are nutritionally dense. Processed foods are nutritionally devoid. When you feel a hunger pang, it's your body's way of saying "I need food", or in other words, nutrients. Eating processed foods is like putting coffee in your car's fuel tank – hey, it's still a liquid, isn't it? Similarly, when you're thirsty it's your body's way of saying "I need water". Rarely do you need more than one glass of water to quench your thirst. However, if you tried to satisfy your thirst with wine or beer it would take a lot more. Water is pure and natural so it instantly feeds your cells; processed drinks are false and clog them. In a nutritional sense they are useless.

Which brings us to the next side effect: **water content**. The low water content alone is a major reason to avoid processed foods. Low water content means low energy. Lack of water means digestion is slowed down by the clogging effect. In order to deal with this, your body ingeniously turns off your energy while providing energy for digestion. This is why people who mainly eat processed food suffer from fatigue, bloating, weight gain, constipation and poor digestion. Processed foods are dead foods. Is this what you want to put into your body?

Thirdly, and the most compelling reason of all for not eating processed foods, are the **man-made, addictive chemicals** that are added to them. There are too many to mention right now, but basically these additives are chemicals and are not designed for human consumption. Evidence is now emerging that not only do they cause disease, but many of them are also designed by the food industry to actually make you fat. After all, fat people eat more food. More food means more sales. And more sales mean more profits for the shareholders. Simple!

Be convinced. Profit is the number one priority of these organisations. In fact, it's probably the only priority. Your health is way down the pecking order. An example is the sweeteners added to low fat and diet foods that we've looked at earlier. They actually make you store fat and crave sugar. Before the introduction of processed foods, we Brits as a nation were fit, slim and healthy. Many of today's diseases were not around even 40 years ago. I believe processed foods are one of the biggest contributors to the current epidemic of obesity worldwide. Please do your best to avoid them whenever possible.

■ CUT THE CRAP PROCESSED FOOD

> ➤ **The easiest way to cut out processed food? Increase the amount of fresh food you eat!**
> ➤ **Don't focus on what you can't have and what's bad for you. Instead, focus on what you can have and what's good for you.**

···➤ *Additives are addictives*

Low fat diets are get fat diets

FOR DECADES NOW, WE'VE BEEN ADVISED TO SLASH THE fat from our diet. It all seemed to make perfect sense at first. We were brainwashed to believe fat makes us fatter. Well, doesn't it? Wrong! Low fat diets are insanity. Since we have all been conned into believing that a low fat diet is best, the food industry has jumped on the bandwagon and made every food possible low fat. They even make foods that were already low fat, such as yoghurts, even lower fat.

The problem is it doesn't work and we are getting fatter and fatter. In fact, most of the clients I see have been battling with a low fat diet only to find their girths getting bigger. We haven't really successfully reduced our fat at all. From 1980-1991 our fat intake remained pretty much the same as it began, around 81 grams a day per person. We then compensated for the fat that we thought we'd cut out by increasing the carbohydrates and animal proteins we ate. We did manage to cut the percentage of calories from fat slightly, but only because we increased the number of calories we ate each day.

Worse, the sugary foods we started loading up on are all acidic. Fat burns fat, and without the correct fat the body literally falls apart. Your metabolic rate slows down, your appetite increases and you seek the fat unknowingly in food such as cakes, biscuits, crisps and chocolate. Yet these all contain the wrong fats. People go out of their way to avoid, butter, cream and oil, and then gorge on fast, convenience foods to satisfy their craving. Madness.

If you have ever wondered why you crave sugary foods after a meal, it's the lack of good fats in your diet. Below you'll find some good fat foods to include in your daily diet. Diets too low in fat have been linked to depression and mood disorders, heart disease, skin problems, brittle nails and, of course, obesity. Naturally low fat foods are good; unnaturally low fat foods are bad.

To sum up, there are healthy fats and unhealthy fats. Make it your business to know which ones to avoid.

Trans fats. Definitely off the menu

These fats are man-made and found in processed foods such as pastry, cakes, biscuits, takeaways, fast foods and many packaged foods. The most common are hydrogenated and partially hydrogenated oils.

Trans fats will without question make you overweight. In addition, they lead to heart disease, cancer, arthritis and diabetes. Believe me, they are killers. They are loaded with calories and junk, and clog up your body. Imagine a lump of lard working its way through your arteries and covering your heart; now you get the picture.

Saturated fat should also be avoided. Mostly derived from animal sources such as dairy meat, poultry and eggs, it contains high levels of cholesterol.

■ CUT THE CRAP **TRANS FATS**

> ➤ **Check the ingredients list on food in the supermarket.**
> ➤ **Under no circumstances buy it if you find any trans fats.**

Margarine - not the healthy alternative

Do you remember all the hype about margarines and how they were supposed to lower cholesterol? Food manufacturers made a big mistake when they sold us that lie. It turned out margarine actually lowered our good cholesterol and increased our bad.

Margarines were originally produced in the late 18th century as a cheap alternative to butter. In the 19th century, food manufacturers cottoned on to the fact that if they made false health claims telling us the "benefits" of eating this synthetic grease, they could sell more. It worked, and there was a nationwide switch to margarines almost overnight.

To this day, they are still trying to hoodwink us, fortifying their products with vitamin D, polyunsaturated, and omega 3s - the exact nutrients that are already present in natural butter. If margarine is supposed to be so healthy, why do they need to fortify it anyway? I am not promoting butter, but eaten in moderation is a "better than" choice.

Stay away from foods that are fortified. In the first place they are out of a carton, and in the second they must have been pretty crap in the first place if they need fortifying

So, margarine may be free of cholesterol, but it increases cholesterol because it is a potent source of trans-fatty acids. Studies have shown that women who ate four or more teaspoons of margarine a day had a 66% greater chance of cardiovascular disease than women who ate about one teaspoon per month. Also, women who eat trans-fatty acids found in margarine and shortening have a much greater risk of contracting breast cancer, the number one killer in women. When men eat this type of fat, they greatly increase their risk of prostate cancer. Do you need any more reasons to give this grease a miss?

Try hummus as an alternative spread. Better still, avoid the bread and you kill two birds with one stone!

···➤ *"Don't eat anything your great-great-grandmother wouldn't recognize as food."* Michael Pollan

High fructose corn syrup – highly unsuitable

These man-made, super-processed sugars play havoc with your body and overtax your hypothalamus, the gland that controls your metabolic rate. They make you fat, unhealthy and crave sugar. They raise insulin levels in your body and encourage it to store fat, particularly around the abdomen. Start reading food labels and you will be surprised where they are hidden.

■ CUT THE CRAP LOW FAT, HIGH FRUCTOSE

- ➤ When shopping, make sure you read the food labels.
- ➤ Don't buy anything that says high fructose corn syrup, corn syrup, sucrose, dextrose or malto dextrose.

···➤ *Many things in life are out of our control, but putting your hand to your mouth isn't one of them!*

Fast foods – fast fat!

You'd have to have lived on Mars not to know that fast food can be fattening. But did you know that the average calorie intake when eating a meal at a fast food restaurant is now 3,500 calories?

Please avoid these foods whenever possible, unless you

know their source, all the added ingredients and how they were prepared. The fast food industry is the fastest way of all to get fat. Many of their products, particularly those from regional and national chains, are literally loaded with calories, saturated fat, trans fats, preservatives, high processed sugars, sweeteners, MSG and nitrates.

Meat, dairy foods and poultry are loaded with growth hormones, antibiotics and drugs. A lot of these foods have also been microwaved and irradiated.

They are often partially or fully cooked prior and then reheated, destroying any nutrients that may have survived at the first bout of cooking. They have little or no fibre, and have been super-refined. The result of all of this processing is an overtaxed hypothalamus, which increases your hunger and makes you physically addicted. It also leads to obesity and depression.

Did you watch that movie, *Supersize Me*? If not, I suggest you do; it's a real eye opener. It followed the fortunes of a man who ate nothing but McDonald's for 30 days straight. At the end of the 30 days, he was hardly recognisable as he had gained a whopping 28lbs! Yes, two stone!

In addition, his blood pressure, triglycerides and cholesterol were sky high and he was considered to be dangerously unhealthy.

This man had been at the peak of physical fitness before he walked through the door of McDonalds. To compound the weight gain, he had also become moody, irritable, constipated, bloated, exhausted and, something he had never been before, depressed. And you thought you had problems! Luckily, at the end of the experiment, with the help of his vegan chef girlfriend he was able to lose the weight and reverse the damage to his health. There was one thing he couldn't lose, however. Can you guess? Yes, the addiction to McDonalds!

Don't ever underestimate the lengths food companies will go to in order to get you addicted. They plan it carefully. There are thousands of food-like products hitting our shelves every year, most of them including new and improved additives. Don't say you haven't been warned!

···➤ *Fast food restaurants were not around 40 years ago.*
Neither was mass obesity.

■ **CUT THE CRAP FAST FOOD**

➤ Instead of going to a fast food restaurant, go
somewhere where they have an open kitchen and
make the pizzas fresh.

➤ Good Chinese and Thai food is generally fresh and
healthy, just go easy on the rice and instead order
vegetables, bean sprouts and salad.

➤ Always order a big side salad.

➤ There's always an alternative to fast food restaurants,
so get wise and stop being a sheep.

➤ Don't be afraid to order "off piste"; in my experience,
waiters are only too happy to help me create a meal
of my choice.

Alcohol – you must beat the booze

Basically a bi-product of purification and decay, alcohol is a
highly acidic substance. It causes increased insulin levels and a
massive strain on your liver and internal organs. Although the
calorific value of alcohol can be quite low, it is still extremely
fattening. In order to neutralise the acid, your body automati-
cally goes into fat storing mode, which means you pile on the
pounds. For these and many other reasons, I recommend you
avoid alcohol whenever possible.

Alcohol's strongly acidic effect also contributes to blood
sugar imbalances, fatigue, premature ageing and obesity.
Drinking alcohol with food slows down your digestion and
causes fermentation and weight gain. So give that drink with
your meal a miss from now on, too.

Alcohol is also a sugar. Readily absorbed, it turns to acid
within hours of you drinking it. As soon as alcohol hits your
stomach it penetrates the walls. That fuzzy feeling you have
is your brains frying, with hundreds of brain cells destroyed.

Those brain cells are never replaced, so no wonder alcohol is linked to memory loss as well. For good measure – no pun intended – alcohol also thins the skin, causes puffiness and promotes premature ageing, just like refined sugar.

The average glass of wine has 250-350 calories, so just two glasses a day can result in 1lb of fat per week, 4lbs a month and 48lbs a year! Personally, I don't think it's worth that penalty.

We used to only drink alcohol on special occasions; now it seems we drink it on any old occasion. Like coffee, tea and many other drinks, it's the habit rather than the substance that makes it so attractive. I always recommend you drink alcohol when you need to, for example when you are socialising or celebrating, but try not to drink in the week when you're just sitting in at home. It will not only slow down your weight loss, but also slow you down too.

One final word of warning. The healthier you become, the less tolerant of alcohol you become. That's normal, so don't worry. But if you don't get hangovers anymore, it's because your liver is shot. Make an appointment today to take a liver function test.

■ **CUT THE CRAP ALCOHOL**

➤ Other people don't usually care how much you're drinking, just that you have a glass in your hand when they do.

➤ So be clever, drink slowly and drink water in between each glass to dilute it.

➤ As you get healthier and your blood becomes more alkaline, try switching to a longer, less sugary drink such as vodka with fresh lime and soda.

Pasta, bread and refined carbohydrates: glue and goo foods

It may surprise you, but all these are overrated. They have

little nutritional value and many processed varieties contain high percentages of refined sugar. Refining and bleaching depletes them of 70% of their vitamin and 90% of their mineral content. Think about it. We used to use pasta mix to hang wallpaper - it's very sticky and clogging!

Bread contains gluten and yeast, which makes it very difficult to digest. It takes approximately eight hours to digest a single slice of bread. During this time, any other food you've eaten will be stuck in your body, causing an energy slump and promoting weight gain. As well as poor digestion, bread also causes bloating and flatulence, while white bread contains no nutrients and is high in sugar. Bread and pasta absorb water and make us bloated within minutes of eating them.

They block the passage for all the other food you eat to be transported down, in effect making everything else fattening too.

If you still want to eat bread, choose wholemeal or granary and lightly toast it to break down the gluten. Don't be fooled by brown bread, it's just white bread dyed brown; the same goes for sugar, both are completely useless when it comes to nutrition. Yet another con by the food industry, they make it brown so we think it must be healthy. Alternatives include wholemeal or seeded tortillas and wholemeal pita.

Sprouted bread is available from most health stores; it tastes a bit like cake and comes in lots of wonderful flavours, carrot and raisin being my favourite. It is delicious and easily digested. I thoroughly recommend it to accelerate fat burning and weight loss.

Diabetics should avoid pasta and bread like the plague, as they can contain as much added sugar as sweet foods. Whilst I'm on the subject, diabetics should avoid a high carbohydrate diet at all costs. All carbohydrates convert to sugar and elevate insulin levels.

Sugar is disguised in so many ways! If you suffer from any inflammatory conditions such as arthritis, I also recommend you cut bread out totally. The yeast aggravates the condition. Give all types of bread a miss for just one week and your discomfort will be alleviated.

■ **CUT THE CRAP BREAD AND PASTA**

➤ Try basmati rice, brown rice, spinach, spelt, corn or soya pastas, all available in health shops.

➤ If you want to eat pasta when you are out, order a starter portion with a vegetable sauce and big salad on the side.

➤ Experiment with wholemeal pita and seeded tortillas, fill them with hummus and avocado salad: absolutely, satisfyingly delicious!

Give long shelf life short shrift

Long life foods have been highly processed, which means not only are they acidic but also lack vitamins and minerals. The nutritional value is virtually destroyed in the process of preserving and therefore they should be avoided.

Fresh foods should always be your first choice, as they give your body energy and enzymes. Enzymes accelerate elimination and weight loss, give energy and are essential for digestion and the absorption of nutrients. Think enzymes, think electricity. Processed foods, however, do not contain enzymes, making them extremely difficult to digest. Proper digestion is also disrupted by the use of condiments, vinegar, alcohol, tobacco, soft drinks, tea, coffee and iced drinks and, of course, food additives. The minute vinegar hits your stomach, for example, all digestive enzymes are destroyed. Lemon or lime juice is a super alternative to vinegar or dressings.

By the way, the sell by date usually has no relation to the food inside the jar or tin. The last thing the food industry would want you to do is keep food longer than they decide. After all, how would they make a profit? In short, the sell by date is a load of crap. These foods are devoid of all enzymes and stripped bare. I hate to tell you, but the array of added chemicals means your tinned and processed foods will probably last longer than you do!

■ **CUT THE CRAP LONG SHELF LIVES**

> ➤ The exception to the rule is tinned fish, but always buy in sunflower or olive oil. Leave brine in the briny!
> ➤ Tinned vegetables and tomatoes are good for convenience and cooking, providing they are only soaked in their own juice. They may still have some nutrients but will be devoid of enzymes so don't forget your salad.
> ➤ Diet foods: need I say more?

Microwaving – made for ageing

If you want to age faster, keep using your microwave. When I read the scientific research behind these things, I immediately cut the plug off mine, told the kids it was broken and haven't used it since. Cooking food in one of these cancer promoters causes premature ageing and damages free radicals and every cell in your body.

Are you sure the waves stop cooking as soon as you open the door? What if they continue to cook as you swallow and then start to penetrate your body? Well, there's a very good chance they do. The superheating effect changes the molecular structure of the food, which in turn causes damage to all your organs. Red and white blood cells deteriorate, cholesterol rises and your immune system is weakened. We used to have a television in the kitchen opposite the microwave, it went mad when we were cooking. I wondered what else those rays were cooking; if you're going to continue microwaving, stand out of the way whilst its on.

The incidence of stomach cancer has been linked to microwaves, thought to be due to the fact that microwaving meat is cancer forming. The evidence to substantiate these studies has resulted in paediatricians no longer advising mothers to use microwaves as a means of heating up infant milk. My advice is to do like I did and cut the plug off!

If you doubt what I'm telling you, try this experiment – and if you must continue to use your microwave, just do it occasionally. Please.

■ CUT THE CRAP MICROWAVING

- ➤ Go to the garden centre and buy two identical plants.
- ➤ Feed one with normal tap water and the other with cooled water which has been heated in the microwave.
- ➤ I have done this three times. The longest my microwave fed plant lasted was 17 days. The others grew beautifully and still flourish! Please try this experiment, the result speak louder than words.

Salt!

Over 20,000 tons of white, refined salt is added to our food each year. We don't need it and it's literally killing us.

Salt will slow down weight loss, cause water retention, bloating and excess thirst. Then there's high blood pressure to top the list, which really puts us at risk of a heart attack. I know people who don't even taste their food before they put the table salt on; how do they know they need it?

They don't – they are either addicted to the stuff or it's a habit. Either way, if you want health and a slender body, salt needs to go.

Don't worry about where you will get your salt from if you don't add it, it's hidden in all labeled foods so you won't go short even if you try.

The only way to eliminate refined salt completely is to stop buying foods with a label and only eat natural.

Now I'm an optimist, but I'm also a realist and it's unlikely that you are going to do that, so you will still get salt from various sources.

To replace salt just use a squeeze of fresh lemon; it does the trick and it's nutritional.

Smoking – sugar here too

Regular smoking can take up to 14 years off your life. Cigarettes are pure acid and the tobacco is roasted in sugar, which makes it even worse. It is impossible to have good health whilst smoking. I offer an excellent smoking cessation programme that I've used with great success for the past nine years with over a 95% success rate and a back up guarantee. The only thing you have to lose is the habit. More information is available on my website.

THESE ARE
A FEW OF MY
FAVOURITE THINGS

OF THE EDIBLE VARIETY, THAT IS. NOTHING TO DO WITH "raindrops on roses and whiskers on kittens", I'm afraid! In truth, there's a whole range of delicious foods out there just waiting for you to discover, or at least renew your acquaintance. As the title says, here are some of my firm favourites to get you going, but I'm sure you'll find many more of your own. Remember to try to shop locally whenever possible, though. The closer you are to a food source, the healthier it is.

···➤ *Almost any foods that originate from the ground*

Great place to start! The golden rule is: if you can pick it or pull it, the chances are you can eat it. Practically all fresh foods are yours for the taking. However, if your goal is to lose weight I would suggest you use white potatoes sparingly. Better still, swap them for sweet potatoes.

Believe it or not, sweet potatoes and butternut squash are much lower in natural sugar. Also, avoid green peppers because they are simply unripe. Farmers give cooked potatoes to pigs to fatten them up to increase commercial value; potatoes may be healthy but they will fatten you up too if you eat too many.

Nuts, seeds and legumes

Nuts and seeds are loaded with protein and calcium, so you simply must include them in your daily diet. This is especially true if you're going to reduce your consumption of animal flesh, which I strongly advise. Sesame seeds have the highest calcium value of any food on this planet, which makes them the ideal supplement if you're also going to reduce your dairy (not that dairy has much calcium in it anyway).

Sprinkle on salads and vegetables, or eat as an afternoon snack. I recommend a small handful a day, about the size of a ping-pong ball. Almonds are particularly good as they are tasty and provide lots of energy. I soak mine overnight, drain the water and then keep them in the fridge.

This makes them much more digestible and I enjoy the taste more. All nuts are good, except peanuts. Avoid these unless you're eating them in the raw form straight from their shells. The way they are processed messes up the amino acid chain and makes them carcinogenic.

Be careful when eating cashews, too, as they are loaded in fat and calories. Just have a small amount. Walnuts are good for memory and the prevention of Alzheimer's, that's why they look like a brain. A good idea is to buy a variety of organic nuts and seeds, and mix them together in a jar. Keep the jar out of sight, though, as constant exposure to anything creates desire. This goes for any junk food you have in your house, too – move it to a place you don't frequent.

····➤ *Put a handful of nuts and seeds in a container every morning, then pop them in your bag. This way they're always on hand when you're hungry!*

Watermelon

One of my family's favourite breakfasts. Sprinkle with ground cinnamon, it's so delicious and refreshing. Watermelon has 40% more lypocene than tomatoes, which has been shown to counteract cancer, especially prostate. It's a great source of vitamin C and full of antioxidants to prevent ageing. This last one especially appeals to me! You can juice watermelon with the skin on, it's beautiful.

Breads

Wholemeal pita, wholemeal and seeded tortilla wraps make

great lunches. Fill with hummus, avocado and lots of fresh salad...yum yum! Add sprouted mung beans and bean sprouts for extra enzymes.

Sprouted bread is available from most good health shops and is a bit like a cake. It comes in a variety of flavours including, carrot and raison, rye and ginger. Toasted with a small amount of soya spread, sprouted bread makes a delicious afternoon snack, which children love, too. It's just as appetising cold and plain, though, and ideal for taking to work or on your travels.

One word of warning: because sprouted bread is so fresh, it goes off very quickly and needs to be refrigerated. I buy it in bulk, slice it and individually wrap and freeze each piece. You can then take out a few pieces whenever you need, and keep them in the fridge for up to four days. If ever I need some "comfort" food, this is my first choice. Freezing is good, it doesn't destroy enzymes.

Always remember, when you eat bread, try to not combine it with animal flesh, including fish. Salads and vegetables can be combined with any food group – think of them as neutral.

Hummus

No, it's not fattening; not unless you eat the whole pot, that is. Try to buy organic whenever possible and remember to choose the real thing, not any of the low fat versions. These are high in carbohydrate and sugar and usually contain additives.

Hummus is very versatile and all flavours are delicious. It's also full of good fats, so enjoy without feeling guilty. The only flavour I recommend you limit is caramelised onion, which is very tasty but very high in sugar as well.

Hummus is a great substitute for salad dressings and spreads, and you can spread it inside your avocados. I use hummus almost every day, usually with my lunchtime salads or wraps. For an afternoon snack, I often chop up some carrots and celery and use it as a dip.

By the way, homemade guacamole is as versatile and nutri-

tious as hummus, also a great way to use up your over-ripe
avocados.

···➤ *To stop yourself over-indulging on hummus (or anything else),*
measure an amount onto your plate instead of eating
directly from the pot. A rough measure per day would be a
tablespoon. More or less is fine, depending on your appetite –
just don't eat the whole pot!

Oily fish

Quick, nutritious and satisfying, all fish is good. Oily varieties
such as salmon, tuna, mackerel, crab and sardines are also an
excellent source of EFA's – essential fatty acids – and should
be eaten daily. When buying tinned tuna fish, make sure it's in
either sunflower or olive oil. Brine is diet mentality, you need
the oils. A tin of sardines or mackerel makes a great afternoon
snack.

I particularly like salmon, monkfish, sea bass and tuna. To
spice them, up try marinating in some garlic, chilli and ginger with lime juice before cooking. You can wrap them in foil
and marinate them whilst in the freezer, then take them straight
from the freezer to the oven. I'm all for an easy life. I usually
make up my marinated parcels once a month and then I'm prepared. Don't forget to label them, though! Cooking your fish
this way is quicker than any convenience meal you can buy.

Spices

Black pepper, cayenne, curry powder, chillies and chilli powder, garlic, ginger, nutmeg and cinnamon are all great for
speeding up your metabolic rate. Anything that gets you "hot"
does the job.

Quorn

Although Quorn has been processed, it does not contain
any nasty ingredients and is still a "better than" choice com-

pared to animal flesh. In fact, I love it because it freezes well and cooks very quickly. Quorn is easy to use and can make a wonderful stir-fries, curry, vegetable chilli or lasagna – I use spinach pasta. You can also make shepherd's pie using sweet potatoes as the topping, and serve with vegetables and a huge salad – another of my children's favourites. When I entertain, I always make a big pot of Quorn chilli and serve it with wild rice and a salad. My guests love it and don't know the difference.

Edame soya beans

These are loaded with antioxidants and are also rich in fibre, which helps nudge down cholesterol. Toss them in a salad or add a ginger dressing and eat for your afternoon snack.

Soya products

Again, strictly speaking this is still a processed food, but without all the nasty additives. If you feel the need to replace your dairy intake, this is a much "better than" choice. Soya milks have improved so much over the last few years; my favourites are the So Good range in the UK and the Silk brand in the USA. If you're like me and still like to put something in your tea, soya milk gives it a nice sweet taste. I add a little agave syrup and it tastes wonderful. Soya yoghurts are also rich and creamy, and soya cheese is a good alternative for children.

···➤ *It's the dosage that's the poison. A little of what you fancy does you good.*

Manuka honey

As you may have gathered by now, this is a particular favourite of mine. A natural sweetener, manuka honey has antibacterial and immune system enhancing benefits. In fact, it is now used in hospitals to prevent infection and can be applied directly to open wounds to accelerate healing. I have a motto, "Don't put on your skin what you can't eat". As my mother discovered, Manuka makes a great facemask too.

Agave syrup is another great sweetening alternative. I love to have a little a couple of times a day, in a cup of peppermint or Redbush tea. I find it satisfies my sweet tooth and stops me craving other junk.

Organic and home-made soups

What more can I say, other than that soup is nourishing, comforting, warm, filling and satisfying? Serve with a nice salad to ensure you get your enzymes. When buying organic soup, get into the habit of always checking the ingredients; avoid the cream based ones and blitz the chunky vegetable and lentil varieties. If sugar is on the top row, forget it and choose another brand.

Brown and wild rice

Rice contains dormant enzymes that are only activated when moistened. This is other another example of Mother Nature's ingenious creations.

In Egyptian times, when royalty died they were buried with enough seeds and grains to take them through to the next life. Thousands of years later when the tombs were opened and grains of the rice were planted, they sprouted and grew into healthy rice. Mother Nature figured out how to preserve foods long before we did. Seeds, rice, all grains and nuts should ideally be soaked the night before to release these dormant enzymes. If you follow this simple tip, you will digest everything much more comfortably.

Oh, and always choose brown, wild or basmati rice rather than the white variety, which is processed.

EFA's – Essential Fatty Acids

Not all acid is bad! EFA's – essential fatty acids – are the good guys of the acid world. As their name suggests they are, well,

■ IS THIS YOU?

- ⏢ LOW METABOLIC RATE AND ENERGY LEVELS
- ⏢ POOR DIGESTION AND BLOATING
- ⏢ CONSTIPATION
- ⏢ WEIGHT GAIN
- ⏢ CRAVINGS – ESPECIALLY SUGAR
- ⏢ POOR CONCENTRATION
- ⏢ MEMORY LOSS
- ⏢ DRY SKIN AND BRITTLE, WEAK NAILS
- ⏢ HIGH BLOOD PRESSURE
- ⏢ DRY EYES
- ⏢ DULL HAIR
- ⏢ ARTHRITIS-LIKE JOINT PAIN
- ⏢ MOOD SWINGS
- ⏢ PMT
- ⏢ DEPRESSION
- ⏢ PREMATURE AGEING
- ⏢ HAIR LOSS/ PREMATURE GREYING

essential! Check out the panel above.

If you suffer from two or more of these symptoms, I would advise you to consider taking a good quality EFA supplement, such as a combined Omega three, six and nine capsule. It's also important to increase your consumption of the foods listed below. While you're at it, try sprinkling Udos oil liberally on your vegetables and salads.

Essential fatty acid deficiency affects cells and tissues throughout your body, including your brain. No part of the body can function without them. In fact, without the correct quantity of EFA's, the body literally falls apart.

The good news is that supplementation reverses all the symptoms of deficiency.

How EFA's help your body

- ➤ **Enhanced fat burning – resulting in rapid weight loss**
- ➤ **Decreased fat production and more calories burnt off as heat**
- ➤ **Increased metabolism**

- Suppressed appetite
- Decreased cravings
- Enhancement of major organs
- Strong nails, shiny hair, clear skin
- Slowed down ageing process
- Reversed skin damage
- Elevated moods and increased desire to be active
- Increased energy levels
- Cleansing of the arteries
- Increased detoxification
- Increased stamina and endurance
- Increased fertility
- Reduced bad fats in the blood
- Improved vision
- Improved brain function
- Strengthened immune system

Great sources of essential fatty acids

Good fats will not make you put on weight. Quite the opposite in fact, they actually promote weight loss. Nuts, seeds and avocados should be included in your diet daily as they contain very high amounts of EFA's. As well as the EFA content, nuts and seeds also have essential nutrients and digestible protein. They are particularly high in vitamins A, B, C and E and have important minerals, calcium, magnesium, potassium, zinc, iron and selenium.

Oils are also important, such as olive oil, coconut, flaxseed oil and avocado oil. Do not cook with olive oil, however, as it becomes unstable and acidic when heated – use sunflower, avocado or vegetable oil instead.

YOUR NUTS!

- Almonds
- Brazil nuts
- Pistachios
- Walnuts

- ➤ **Sunflower seeds**
- ➤ **Pumpkin seeds**
- ➤ **Cashews**
- ➤ **Chestnuts**
- ➤ **Flaxseeds**
- ➤ **Linseeds**

Cho Yung Tea

A weight loss tea that Rod Stewart's wife, Penny Lancaster, attributes her weight loss to. I love this tea, it tastes really good and when I drink it I can actually feel my metabolism speeding up. If I need a bit of a lift this is always my first choice; it's a great alternative to coffee and, of course, much healthier. it's high in anti-oxidents and contains no nasty ingredients – a good choice all round in my opinion. I love the fact that it can be drank alone without milk or sweetener and I always keep a couple of sachets in my bag when I'm out and about. I'm sure that if you try it, you will love it!

There, you have some of my favorite foods. Now you need to find your own. We all have a habit of buying the same foods week in and week out, so give yourself a little more time when you next go shopping and explore the other aisles and organic sections. Check out the health food shops, too. Above all, always make it your business to find out exactly what you are eating, and don't trust the manufacturers.

YOU ARE
WHAT YOU DRINK

Up the ante

YOU MUST HAVE HEARD HOW GOOD WATER IS FOR YOU,
so why aren't you drinking it? Let me explain how vital water
is if you want to shed your excess weight and reach outstanding health.

A major component of blood, water flows through the
arteries carrying essential nutrients to cells and flushing away
harmful waste products through the kidneys. Water also
boosts your well-being by helping to restore and revitalise
your body. While you can survive for some time without food,
you can only live a few days without water.

Maintaining fluid levels is essential for the body to function. It helps you absorb vitamins, minerals, natural sugars
and other nutrients, thus speeding up the rate at which glu-
cose is absorbed and boosting energy levels. Drinking pure
water is also vital to aid digestion, ensuring your body receives
essential nutrients and flushing out harmful toxins.

It may come as a surprise, but by the time you're thirsty
you are already dehydrated. It's estimated that 75% of the
UK population is mildly dehydrated; even mild dehydration
can lead to constipation, bad breath, headaches, anxiety, dull-
looking skin, a weakened immune system and disease. It's also
a major contributor to excess body fat.

The average adult loses around two litres of fluid on a
normal day – more in hot weather or during exercise. Fluid
loss occurs whenever water is excreted through the skin and
kidneys and with every exhalation of breath, so it's important
that you replenish fluid regularly. However, a recent survey
shows that most adults don't drink enough water.

Before the introduction of coffee, tea, soda and alcohol,
water was the only drink available. Taste was not the deciding
factor; we drank it for thirst, intuitively knowing our bodies

relied on it for every major function. To be sure you are drinking enough water, check the colour of your urine. It needs to be clear in colour. Yellow urine indicates you are dehydrated. Weight loss is difficult, if not impossible, if you are not drinking enough water. Tea, coffee and cordials are not considered water because of their diuretic affect. Nor are those dubious products that say "naturally flavoured".

As I've said, they are crap, so cut them out. If you want to flavour water, do it yourself. I add cucumber, fresh lemon, lime or strawberry; it takes seconds. The more caffeine you drink, the more water you lose, so watch this too.

■ ARE YOU DEHYDRATED?

There are eight signs of dehydration you need to be aware of:

SIGN	
1	A DRY MOUTH
2	DARK URINE – it should be clear
3	PINCH THE SKIN ON THE BACK OF YOUR HAND – IS IT SLOW TO BOUNCE BACK?
4	PERSISTENT HEADACHES. The brain is 75% water, so hydration improves mental agility and concentration.
5	MOOD SWINGS
6	SUNKEN EYES or DARK CIRCLES AROUND THE EYES
7	BAD BREATH. This is caused by a build-up of bacteria – if you are well hydrated it's flushed out.
8	CONSTIPATION. You must have at least one easy, well-formed stool a day, anything less is a serious sign that your body is in dis-ease.

⋯➤ *Headaches are usually just a symptom of dehydration. So try drinking a glass of water rather than popping a pill next time.*

Hot water is wonderful for supporting your digestion, while cold will have the opposite effect and slow it down. For this reason, I recommend you avoid drinking very cold drinks and drink them at room temperature instead. Carry a bottle of water on your travels wherever you go, too – spring water is the best source of natural minerals. Tap water doesn't contain many essential minerals so for that reason I prefer to buy it by mineral. In some areas tap water contains chlorine, lead, pesticides and herbicides, prescription drugs and pharmaceuticals, all of which present a real danger to your health. There are however, a handful of home filtration units that can remove these substances (activated carbon ones, using a double cartridge).

For that reason I choose bottled. It's a good idea to keep a supply of bottles of water behind your seat in your car, this way you can drink and drive (water only, folks!). Preparation is the key for everything.

···➤ *Water is 30% oxygen!*

Don't get the hump

Unfortunately, we do not have an organ that stores water, so we store it in our fat cells. This is why fat people are rarely thirsty. Every fat cell you have is 70% water and the body likes to hang onto its reserves. This is its built-in, natural reservoir. We used to think a camel's hump was made of water, but now realise that's not exactly true. The hump is filled with fat and the fat contains water.

Every single bodily function relies on water and, as we've seen, you cannot live without it. If you are not drinking enough, your body will preserve its fat cells at all costs. This may be despite the fact that you are dieting or reducing calories. To lose weight, you need to trade fat cells for water. Be warned, though. Initially when you increase your water intake, don't be surprised if you're running to the toilet every 20 minutes. Don't worry, this is normal and great for detoxification. What's happening is that at first your body will not trade with you. It needs to make sure it can trust you to provide fluids on a daily basis. Within seven to 10 days of constant drinking, a trusting relationship forms and your body starts to release the fat cells and increase your thirst. How ingenious it is! It's the most magnificent machine known to man.

You have to persevere until you naturally acquire a thirst. Once you have done this, don't be surprised to find that water will be the only drink that truly satisfies you. You will also reduce acidic drinks naturally. Please avoid carbonated drinks in particular. Carbonated drinks became popular in the seventies with the introduction of soda streams, and ever since we've seen a steady stream of fizz hitting the shelves. Americans are the number one soda pop drinkers in the world; no prizes for guessing who's second.

We also seem to be addicted to drinking our own waste. CO2 is a waste product, yet fizzy drinks are fizzed with C02 – the very thing the body works so hard to excrete. Don't put CO2 back into your body, please. For more convincing, just think: what's the first thing you do when you drink a fizzy drink? Yes, burp! That's because your body is trying to eject the stuff. Once you've bypassed the burp, it hits your stomach and gives you wind. Then you wonder why you're bloated.

Another side effect of these drinks is that when the gas hits your stomach it falsely stimulates your appetite. Drinking fizzy drinks also leaches calcium from the bones, hence the growth in reported cases of paediatric osteoporosis. Not a lot going for them, is there?

Stick with still natural water as Mother Nature intended. Drink water 10 minutes before and after meals, and not during as this dilutes your digestive juices. To work out how much water you actually need, divide your body weight (in lbs) in half - this is how many fluid ounces you need. For example, a man weighing 180lbs would need 90 fl oz of water.

···➤ *Don't drink more than two glasses of water at any one time, it's too hard on your kidneys.*

THE POWER
OF EXERCISE

What you don't use, you lose!

EXERCISE IS NON-NEGOTIABLE! I KNOW YOU DON'T WANT to hear this, but it's another truth you just can't avoid. To achieve the optimum balance of health and fitness, you need to train your metabolism. Remember, your goal is not just to become slim but also fit and healthy. And health is not just the absence of disease.

In order to reach your ideal weight, and most importantly maintain it, you need to exercise. So once you get your diet on track, you need to start moving your butt! I can hear you groaning and moaning already; don't panic just yet, though. You don't have to run out and get a fancy gym membership and flog yourself every day, you just need to get moving more. Encouragingly, research has shown that if you exercise consistently over a 12 month period, you will form this positive addiction for a lifetime.

Before the Second World War, we all were extremely active. Most people didn't own a car and walked on average a minimum of five miles a day. People were fitter and, of course, slimmer in those days. In 1930, less than 1% of the British population was obese. Similarly, before 1905 heart disease and cancer were far less common, yet now they are our biggest killers. The big sugar and flour mills developed around this time and we began to get our first taste of processed foods. Since then we have continued to process our foods. We have continued to eat more. And we have continued, despite great breakthroughs in medical science and the invention of diet foods, to get sicker and fatter. The only thing we haven't continued to do is exercise.

In the old days, people didn't need to join a gym to exercise because that's what they did naturally. It was a normal, everyday function. They didn't have to think about it, they just did it. It was as natural to them as blinking, breathing or swallowing. Mother Nature provided us with limbs so we could move around, not so we could sit in the car, slouch on the settee or lie in bed all morning.

Walk the walk

If you have two legs and can walk, then get walking! Walking is a wonderful, natural activity that is therapeutic as well as physically challenging. Start off by walking for 30 minutes and then build up to an hour a day. I love my daily walks. I do them first thing in the morning, and while out I listen to my audio books, say my affirmations and plan my day ahead. Being outside gives me time to connect with nature, breathe in the fresh air and generally enjoy the great outdoors. The great spiritual gurus tell us how important it is to connect with nature every day; it is very grounding and helps you maintain balance. Unfortunately, as you may have noticed, the sun doesn't shine too often here in the UK, and those cold and rainy days can be somewhat challenging. However, there's no such thing as bad weather, weather is just weather, and with the right clothes you can wrap up and still enjoy being outside.

Do you remember as a child how you used to love jumping in puddles and singing in the rain? Do you recall protesting when you had to put on a coat? I do. We in Britain we have become too obsessed with complaining about the weather. It's become a national pastime and often the first thing people talk about when they meet. And how many people have to check out the weather before they decide what type of day they're going to have? If it's raining in the morning they open the curtains and say, "Another lousy day!" What's lousy about it? Give it a chance; you haven't even started your day yet, so how can you make such a statement? All you have to do is change your outlook to a positive one, put on a hat and coat and you can make that day whatever you want it to be. By the way, this applies to everything else in life too.

I bought a weighted walking vest recently that makes my

walk more challenging and also helps to tone up my legs and butt. At first I found it difficult to walk at my usual pace and felt like a robot. Now, like anything else, it's got easier and easier and I'm adding more weights to increase the resistance. If you want to know more about these vests, they are available on my website. They take walking to another level and really improve your overall fitness.

I also recommend the use of a pedometer, a discreet little device you attach to your waistband that counts the steps as you walk. Aim to do 10,000 steps a day, which will enable you to burn approximately 8lbs of fat a month. The other thing a pedometer does is to help you evaluate your energy expenditure. Most of us haven't got a clue how much energy we use each day and yet we eat roughly the same amount of calories regardless. If one day you have only done say, 2,000 steps, you need to either eat less or get moving more to lose weight. Remember the car metaphor: you wouldn't fill your car if you hadn't done the mileage. The same rule applies to your body.

One of my many success stories is a lady called Barbara, who has reached her goal weight and feels that, in her own words, she's been "reborn". A few weeks ago she called to thank me and told me proudly:

"If I haven't done my 10,000 steps by the evening, I jump in the car and head for the gym. I hop on the treadmill and within no time at all I've achieved my goal!"

Barbara has done this every single day since leaving my office. That's what I call commitment.

Want to lose weight? Lift weights!

Walking, running and aerobic classes are all great cardio workouts, but if you want to burn fat you really need to lift weights. You can lose weight doing aerobic training, but it's unlikely you will reshape your body. For example, if you started out a pear shape you will probably end up a smaller pear shape. You won't have transformed your body, you will just be a smaller version of the original you. For years I did at least four to five aerobic classes a week and never lost weight or changed shape. I certainly felt better, but my primary goals were to lose weight, burn fat and tone up, and cardio is unlikely to achieve these.

Have you ever noticed how you see certain people at the gym every time you go? They always seem to be there, working out for long periods, sweating and battling the bulge. Yet have you also noticed that these people are often still overweight and the same shape? Even the fitness instructors who do three or four classes a day are often overweight or have a wobbly spare tyre. Hours of scientific research have convinced me that such people are over-exercising. This actually stops you burning fat, increases your appetite and takes you further away from your goals.

If you do nothing but aerobic exercise, even if you eat less, your results will not be optimal. Brief, intense periods of exercise produce impressive physical results while at the same time clearing your mind, relieving stress and allowing you to focus on your daily goals. Believe me, you can't beat it.

Building muscle burns fat

The best way to build muscle is to do resistance training three times a week, for a period of approximately 50 minutes. Through resistance training you can significantly increase your metabolic rate and the rate your body burns fat. When you gain muscle, your body requires more energy to maintain this new muscle and therefore you burn calories. Another reason why men can generally eat more than women and lose weight faster is that genetically they have more muscle (just not fair, is it?). Fat, on the other hand, is very different from muscle. It doesn't require any energy at all to maintain it, it just sits there and does nothing but weigh you down.

There's more, too. Not only does weight training gives you the ability to burn fat, it literally transforms, sculpts and re-shapes your body. Even though aerobic exercise can help you burn fat, it often increases your appetite and does not transform the body. Spending hours and hours in the gym isn't productive at all.

Age also comes into the equation. As you grow older, you lose muscle mass. This process begins from around the age of 25, which is when most men and women start seeing their body fat percentage increase. From his early 30s to his mid-60s, the average man's body fat level often doubles from around 18% to 36%. In the same time frame, the average women's body fat can change from 30% to 44%. This is why your metabolic rate drops and you get a spongy, flabby look around your midriff, face, upper arms and back. If you're lucky, your body weight may stay the same but your body shape will change drastically due to the increase in fat and decrease in lean muscle. So for most of us, it's inevitable. We get older, we get fatter, we lose lean muscle mass, we lose strength. When we lose strength, we become weak and fragile, and prone to a whole host of illnesses, disabilities and injuries.

Sounds like something to look forward to, doesn't it? Don't worry, it's not all doom and gloom. By including weight bearing exercises, such as weight lifting or resistance training, into your life, you can build bone density, strength and lean muscle mass. You can also increase your metabolic rate, burn fat and lose weight. Recent university studies have proved that weight training makes a significant contribution to anyone's quality of life, no matter what their age.

It's never too late to start weight training, either. And you don't need any special skill or advanced level of fitness. No matter what your current level of fitness, whether you are a beginner or have been working out for years, if you're healthy then you're ready to pick up some weights right now.

When starting, you have two basic options. You can purchase some weights to use at home, or you can join a gym. I prefer to go to the gym as I find it more motivating, but it's your choice. If you decide to get your own kit, try looking in the second hand section of the newspaper or on eBay. You will find literally hundreds of items of secondhand home exercise equipment. This isn't because the owners have become super fit and achieved their goals, rather, it's usually because the equipment has become a clothes hanger or a dust gatherer. You need to be highly motivated and disciplined to work out at home.

I always recommend working out three times a week, preferably first thing in the morning. I call it RPE: rise, pee and exercise. This is the time of the day when your energy is high, you're well rested and have no other distractions. Also, it sets you up for high calorie burning throughout the day, while the release of feel good chemicals make you feel great! I pack my gym stuff the night before and set my alarm away from the bed so I have to get up. Once I'm up, I meditate, walk my dog and then exercise. Everyone else in the house is asleep, so there are no distractions and I don't feel that anyone is being neglected. I love the peace and quiet and the time for myself; it's a perfect way to start the day. Before you start out have a few sips of water and then take a bottle with you to keep you fully hydrated.

Personally, I have never been able to exercise in the evening. There's always something that gets in the way, and this is the time my energy is at its lowest. In the evening, it's simply too easy to think of an excuse not to exercise. In the winter months it can sometimes be challenging to get my butt out of a warm, cosy bed, but nowhere near as challenging as dealing with a weight issue.

A note of caution. When training, it's important that you never work the same muscles two days consecutively. This is a common mistake and the main reason people find it difficult to achieve muscle definition. Muscles grow while you rest, not while you are working out. Working out is effectively damaging the muscle; the rest period repairs it and a scar forms over the muscle, giving it more size. If you don't rest your muscles for at least 24 hours, they can't cannot recover or grow in size. Bill Phillips, author of Body for Life, uses the following excellent analogy:

"Imagine a muscle cell as a structure, a building. And imagine exercise as a slight earthquake. After the tremor causes structural damage to the building, a repair team has to come in and rebuild it."

Essentially, this is what happens after an effective free-weight work out: you slightly damage the muscle cells, then your body mobilises to fix the damage. This repair work requires energy that, under the right circumstances, will be pulled from your stored body fat. This is another reason why effective weight training helps you burn fat. Imagine that the rebuilding workforce were in the process of putting that house back together. They were almost done when, lo and behold, another earthquake hit! Obviously, the further damage done by the earthquake would make it weaker, not stronger.

Give yourself a break

The message here is that without proper rest between workouts, your muscles cannot grow properly. Over-exercising of any description has the reverse of the desired effect. This also goes for the time you spend doing your actual workout. After around 45 minutes of intense exercise, your body starts to work against itself and use muscle for energy.

So keep your sessions brief and precise, no more than 50 minutes. Don't stand chatting, just get on with your workout and go home. In between workouts, allow yourself time to rest and relax. As well as proper nutrition, make sure you get plenty of sleep – I recommend eight hours every evening. This is the time when your body rejuvenates and repairs itself and is very important.

I also suggest you leave a gap of four hours between eating your last meal and bedtime. The optimum time to go to sleep is between 10.00 and 10.30pm. Universal energy is low, the birds are asleep and there is stillness in the air. Your metabolic rate has dropped and digestion is switched off. Going to bed at this time will enable you to follow the rhythms of nature.

In the same vein, the ideal time to rise is between 6.00 and 6.30 in the morning. The energy of the universe is high, the birds are singing and nature is awakening. As I've said, this is my favorite time of day. I just love the mornings; the stillness feels sacred. If you are one of those people who get up at the last minute and rushes around like an idiot, experiment with setting your alarm an hour earlier. Waking up earlier not only gives you more energy but also increases your calorie burning power. I guarantee that after only a few days, you'll feel so much more relaxed and organised– both very empowering feelings.

Another big help for burning fat is to exercise on an empty stomach, then leave an hour before you eat anything. For general health, fitness and muscle-building, I recommend you have a light breakfast, such as fruit, prior to exercising, and then a high protein snack such as a Spirulina soya shake, a small banana, an apple or a few almonds within 20 minutes of finishing.

Have fun

With exercise, the most important thing is to find something you enjoy. Doing an exercise you don't enjoy is pointless. As well as being a chore, the negativity just creates an influx of cortisol that encourages your body to store fat and break-down muscle.

So if weight training doesn't appeal to you, try salsa or ashtanga yoga. If you want to do a class, have a go at body pump or circuit training, both great for burning fat and building muscle.

I schedule my training in my diary like an appointment and I suggest you do the same. Nothing – and I mean nothing, apart from life and death – can move it. I like to exercise three times a week: Mondays, Wednesdays and Fridays. On Tuesday and Thursday I do some light aerobic exercise such as a power walk, a bike ride or a gentle jog. Generally, I'm more relaxed about the weekends, sometimes just resting, sometimes walking or doing a yoga class.

Now, I'm in no way fanatical about exercise, and I certainly don't have a body like Madonna (I wish!). For my age, though, I think I look pretty good. I exercise for health and vitality. If I applied more discipline and intensity, I'm sure I could achieve the body of my dreams, but enjoying balance in my life is more of a priority than the size of my biceps. I suspect you feel the same.

If your lifestyle doesn't allow you to train in the morning, keep your gym kit in the car and go straight from work. From what I've seen, going home first means you probably won't make it.

Good vibrations

Many people tell me they hate exercising altogether. My response to this is, "Do you hate it more than you hate being fat, tired and sick?" Usually they say no.

However, if you are one of those who loathe being overweight, but can't bear the thought of the gym either, then you're in luck. You now have another option. A new concept in physical training, which you can do in the comfort of your own home. In fact, it's great for the whole family and takes a quarter of the time of an average workout.

What on earth am I talking about? Vibration training. It's all the rage at the moment. Ask Madonna or the whole host of celebs, Premier League footballers and WAGs who use it!

In truth, vibration training has been available for some time, but was originally developed for astronauts in the 70s and used exclusively by wealthy celebrities and specialised private clinics around the world. Today, as with everything, the price has come right down and this new concept is literally sweeping the country.

What I love is how simple and easy the equipment is to use, and how effective the results are. In just 15 minutes a day you can transform the shape of your body. You can get a whole body workout and stretch, tone and build your muscles. Now that's my kind of exercise! The other thing I love is that the equipment is pleasing on the eye and blends well in my living room. If you want to know more, you'll find full details on my website. This type of accelerated training definitely achieves maximum results in the minimum of time.

So remember, find something you like and start moving now. The rewards are life giving. It doesn't matter what place you're coming from, all that matters is where you are going.

Treat yourself to a massage day

> ➤ Create a new daily ritual of self-massage, use a body brush prior to showering to stimulate lymphatic drainage.
> ➤ After you've showered, massage your body with a pure, unrefined oil such as almond or sesame oil.
> ➤ Repeat the following either out loud or mentally:
>> *I love every cell in my body!*
>> *I love every cell in my arms!*
>> *I love every cell in my legs!*
>> *I love every cell in my stomach!*
>> *I love every cell in my buttocks!*

YOUR
PERSONAL
TRANSFORMATION

"Be the change you want to see in the world."

GHANDI

ARE YOU READY TO GET STARTED? IS THIS THE TIME TO transform your life? Do you wish to create the health, energy and slender body you deserve? Is it time to truly *Cut The Crap*?

It's **yes**, **yes**, **yes** and **yes** again, I hope!

By now, you have the full toolbox. You've got everything you need to create a healthy lifestyle and reach your ideal weight. There's an abundance of healthy food just waiting for you out there, so you need never be bored or hungry. Simply focus on the foods that create energy and rebalance your body and you will naturally be drawn towards healthy choices and away from processed crap.

As I said at the beginning, though, nothing is banned (except sweeteners). You can literally eat what you want, when you want. Now you know the consequences of eating processed foods, you can make an intelligent choice and go for what nourishes your body. Although I hope you're changing your mind about the things you once called your favourites.

To recap, this is not a diet for you to fail at. We're all human and from time to time it's natural to lapse. If you eat something "out of range", as long as you enjoyed it, don't beat yourself up. However, if you didn't even enjoy it, you have my permission to go ahead and give yourself a kicking! Eating food we don't like is a waste of calories and, most of all, a waste of energy.

If you do stray, whatever you do, don't quit. You've done that too many times before, that's why you are here. Too many people pack in because of one moment of weakness. Never let a lapse become a collapse. Life is to be enjoyed, so make your journey an enjoyable one and stop aiming for perfection.

In truth, this is just a beginning of a process, a new way of thinking and eating for the rest of your life. There is no rush, so just take it easy. Quick fixes are not the answer, as you already know. Take baby steps along the way and you will eventually reach your goal. Implement small changes weekly and allow the process to unfold naturally. It took me over two years to lose my weight and I have never put a pound back on again. Your mind has to understand the process. Changes need to become new habits, both mentally and physically. Your stomach and skin need to shrink slowly, and you need to live and be happy while they do.

Experiment with new foods and recipes, and find or create a food plan that suits you and which you thoroughly enjoy. I've made some suggestions and recommendations that have worked for many of my clients, but we are all individuals and ultimately you have to find what works for you. I have a client who lost five stones and has her main meal for breakfast and her breakfast for dinner!

I remember when I did the slimming club thing; if I lost weight I used to go home and reward myself with food. I used to overeat and then regain some of the lost weight again. How stupid I was. I wasn't rewarding myself, I was punishing myself. The reward is not food, it's the gift you give yourself by increasing your chances of survival. My healthy, vibrant body makes me feel happier than any taste of food or chocolate could ever do, and it does it 24 hours a day.

Remember, too, that it's as important to change your psychology as the food you eat. Start each day with your personal affirmation, e.g. "Every day in every way I am getting slimmer and slimmer". Repeat this at least 20 times, and do it with emotion. The more you use positive affirmations, the more your subconscious mind will become programmed to creating the new, slimmer you. Instead of asking yourself negative questions such as "Why am I so fat?" ask yourself a positive one such as "How do I get slim?" or "What do I want to look like?" Everything in life begins with a thought; the only difference between successful people and those who fail is their mindset. As part of the process of eliminating negative thoughts, delete the word "diet" from your vocabulary and start to act and think like someone who is already slim. Put a slim photo where you can see it and visualise yourself like that daily. Start to filter the crap from your life. Read food labels and become aware of what you are actually eating.

Listen to your body. It will always tell you what you need, as long as you take the time to listen. Connect with your body by loving and accepting it. After all, how can you change a body that you're disconnected from? It's like making a phone call with your phone unplugged. Every cell in your body responds to messages from your brain. The more you practise self-awareness, the easier your weight loss will be.

Make sure you try the massage routine. It may feel a little strange at first, especially when you touch areas of your body you don't like or have avoided looking at in the past. Remember, repetition is the mother of skills. The more you practice, the easier it will be. To change, you need to make friends with your body; after all it's the only body you've got. To nourish your body you need to love it first. If you dislike it, it's easy to punish it, yet thankfully it's hard to abuse something you love.

In truth, loving yourself is the first and most important change to enable you to lose weight. Over-eating, eating poisons, smoking, over-consumption of alcohol and self-criticism are all forms of escapism and self-abuse. These actions merely sabotage your life and result in low self-esteem and feelings of weakness.

Finally, I cannot over-estimate the importance of exercise as part of your new healthy lifestyle. It's also vital that you find something you enjoy. As you begin to experience all the positive benefits of making changes, you will be eager to make even more. Don't ever forget that you can be whatever you resolve to be. Decide to be something in this world and you will be something. "I cannot" never accomplished anything. "I will try" works wonders.

Welcome back to the house of health! I hope I get the opportunity to meet you personally one day.

The power of Energised Greens

I couldn't finish this book without telling you about a wonderful superfood drink I discovered over 15 years ago. For those of you who respect the importance of alkalising your body, but think you may struggle to eat the necessary amount of fruits, vegetables and other live foods, this may be a quick and easy solution.

Green drinks are like green foods, probably one of the most nutritionally dense and food supplements available. These superfoods contain a vast array of green foods, fruits and grasses to ensure you get your more than your daily quota. They come in a powder form that is easily mixed with water. The main benefits are health, energy and weight loss, but the list goes on and on. They are right up there on the Ph scale, somewhere around 15, which makes them extremely alkalising. Because they are liquid, penetrate your cells quickly, they can be used as a great quick start for your new, healthy lifestyle.

Although I do my best to make 70% of my diet fresh, live foods, some days are better than others so my green drink is my insurance policy. Just one serving is equivalent to over 4lbs of vegetables – which is pretty impressive! I aim to have a least two servings, sometimes three, per day. When I started my weight loss journey, I took up to five a day. I carry my green drink with me and sip it continuously throughout the day; I call it my holy grail.

There are lots of green drinks on the market and most of them taste ghastly. Energised Greens is different; as well as being a superior product it tastes very pleasant and is easy to mix. I love my green drinks and can't imagine my life without them. I drink it first thing in the morning and when I'm exercising instead of water. Of course I am not advocating replacing fresh, live foods, but as an addition and back up I think this works well.

> **For more information on Energised Greens and other alkalising products, go to www.energisedgreens.com**
> **For daily health and weight loss tips, follow Deborah on Twitter @1cutthecrap**

■ THE ULTIMATE DETOX AND WEIGHT LOSS RETREAT

AN INVITATION TO SURRENDER

An opportunity to relax, rejuvenate and lose weight. Educational, inspirational with guaranteed results!

···➤ Life changing in every sense: lose your weight and change your eating and thinking habits whilst immersing yourself in an inward journey of self awareness.

···➤ Relax in the luxurious surroundings and rediscover your true, thinner self.

···➤ Remove unwanted eating habits and let Deborah teach you the secrets to long term health and weight management.

···➤ With average weight loss of 7-10lbs, you will be energised and remotivated.

···➤ If you are serious about your health, this is an opportunity not to be missed.

IF YOU WOULD LIKE TO JOIN DEBORAH
AT ONE OF HER WEIGHT LOSS RETREATS IN THE UK
OR ABROAD

Call 0845 330 1367
or
Log onto www.ayurveda4life.co.uk

■ APPENDICES

GOOD SOURCES OF:

Proteins
- Beans
- Bean sprouts
- Soya milk
- Seeds, nuts
- Fish – all types
- Lentils
- Tofu
- Whole grains
- Hummus

Good fats EFAs *(essential fatty acids) – essential for brain and nerve function. Vital to get lots of*
- Omega 3
- Seeds – especially flaxseeds
- Rapeseed oil
- Avocado oil
- Avocados
- Nuts – especially almonds and hazelnuts
- Oily fish
- Soya milk and yoghurt
- Linseed oil
- Olive oil
- Green leafy vegetables
- Hummus

Carbohydrates *For energy use complex carbohydrates – avoid sugar and white flour*
- Wholegrain rice
- Wholemeal pita bread
- Oats
- Granary bread
- Sprouted bread
- Beans and lentils

Fibre *Vital for health – keeps bowels healthy, lowers cholesterol and regulates appetite.*
- Whole grains
- Fruit and vegetables
- Beans and lentils
- Nuts and seeds

Iron *Used in production of red blood cells and oxygen transportation. Best absorbed with Vitamin C.*
- Green leafy vegetables, e.g. kale cabbage
- Beans and lentils
- Pumpkin seeds
- Figs and dates
- Tofu
- Millet
- Dried apricots

Calcium *For teeth, bones and muscles. Also for hormones and blood clotting. Plant sources are very useful.*
- Green leafy vegetables, e.g. kale, spinach, watercress
- Broccoli
- Almonds
- Swede
- Tofu (calcium set)
- Soya milk and yoghurts (fortified)
- Sunflower seeds (one of the highest)
- Spouted seeds
- Mung beans
- Bean sprouts

Iodine *Important for metabolism and healthy functioning of thyroid gland. Ensure good supply.*
- Green leafy vegetables
- Asparagus
- Kelp (kombu) – dried or tablets

Magnesium *For bone strength, nerve and muscle function.*
- Green leafy vegetables
- Whole grains
- Soya beans
- Apples
- Cashew nuts
- Almonds
- Avocados, bananas, apricots

Selenium, Phosphorus & Potassium *Selenium is an antioxidant and fights disease. Potassium is for blood pressure and calcium balance.*
- Brazil nuts
- Whole grains
- Chickpeas
- Hummus
- Pumpkin seeds
- Yeast extract
- Strawberries
- Bananas
- Tomatoes
- Many fruits and vegetables

■ **DISCOUNT VOUCHER**

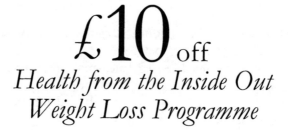

£10 off
Health from the Inside Out
Weight Loss Programme

THE EASY ANSWER TO WEIGHT LOSS

This audio weight loss programme makes weight loss easier than you can ever imagine. From the comfort of your home, whilst driving your car or on the move you can now benefit from this hugely successful concept. Previously only available by private consultation, Deborah will guide and support you through every stage of weight loss and most importantly weight management.

Includes ground breaking nutritional information, your daily eating plan and the added bonus of a self-hypnosis session. If you need to eradicate unwanted eating habits and implement healthy ones, this is the programme for you!

➤ **To order simply call 0845 330 1367 or log onto www.cutthecrap.co.uk**
➤ **Private consultations with Deborah available by email request. info@cut the crap.co.uk**

Lightning Source UK Ltd.
Milton Keynes UK
UKOW041349230512

193143UK00004B/4/P